D1480405

SALESMAN
SURGEON

SALESMAN SURGEON

The Incredible Story
of an Amateur
in the Operating Room

by William MacKay

as told to Maureen Mylander

McGRAW-HILL BOOK COMPANY

New York St. Louis San Francisco
Düsseldorf Mexico Toronto

Book design by Joan E. O'Connor

Copyright © 1978 by William MacKay.
All rights reserved.
Printed in the United States of America.
No part of this publication may be reproduced,
stored in a retrieval system, or transmitted
in any form or by any means, electronic, mechanical,
photocopying, recording, or otherwise, without the
prior written permission of the publisher.

23456789 DO DO 78321098

Library of Congress Cataloging in Publication Data

MacKay, William, 1943-
    Salesman surgeon.

    1. Surgeons—Professional ethics.   2.   MacKay,
William, 1943-   3.   Sales personnel—New York (State)
—Biography.   I. Mylander, Maureen.   II.   Title.
RD27.7.M33   617   78-15631
ISBN 0-07-044390-4

To my wife,
with love and affection

CONTENTS

CONTENTS

INTRODUCTION

I met the author, Bill MacKay, for the first time in the summer of 1977. At that time I was the Assistant Chief of the Suffolk County, New York, District Attorney's Frauds Bureau. I was conducting an investigation into allegations that Bill MacKay, a medical-supply salesman, had performed surgery at the request of doctors in two leading Suffolk County hospitals. I must admit that this first meeting was extremely turbulent. When it ended, I was thoroughly convinced that William MacKay was a liar, a braggart and a charlatan. This opinion was soon to change.

The subject of salesmen performing surgery in Suffolk County was first brought to my attention by Mr. Matthew Lifflander, Counsel and Director of the Medical Practice Task Force, Standing Committee on Health, Assembly of the State of New York. His committee had uncovered at least twelve separate occasions in which Bill MacKay allegedly had performed surgery on Long Island. The source of this information was Bill MacKay himself and for the most part was still uncorroborated. The matter was referred to me for evaluation, investigation, and prosecution, if that be deemed necessary.

After I reviewed each of the twelve instances of surgery through the unsworn testimony of MacKay, I was shocked but still unbelieving. How could a doctor allow this high-school drop-out to participate so intimately in major surgery ranging from implantation of prosthetic devices (hips, knees and ankles) to brain surgery? I was convinced that it had to be a hoax and that I would eventually expose MacKay as a complete fraud.

In order to facilitate my investigation I concentrated on a single case, that of Franklin Mirando. It was a total hip transplant that took place at Smithtown General Hospital in July 1975. The surgeon was Dr. David Lipton. The assistant was Dr. Harold Massoff. This appeared to be the best case to begin with, since, according to MacKay's testimony, there were severe complications that could be verified quickly. If MacKay was telling the truth, his story would be corroborated. If he was lying, this would readily be apparent.

The first step in my investigation was to obtain Franklin Mirando's chart from Smithtown General Hospital. This chart contained detailed information on Mirando's July 1975 operation. It gave me the length of the operation, the names of those who participated in the procedure, and the complications of surgery. The chart immediately verified part of MacKay's story—that is, the operation was extremely long. It was broken into two portions. There was a morning session and an afternoon session. The chart makes it clear that the operation ran from approximately 8:30 A.M. to 6:30 P.M.

The details of the operation, as found in the chart, matched MacKay's recitation almost exactly. How could MacKay know these minute details unless he was present? However, the chart and other hospital records failed to indicate his presence. Why?

From the hospital chart of Franklin Mirando I was able to compose a detailed list of witnesses to the operation. My next step was to conduct interviews. I immediately ran into difficulty. No one would talk to me. I quickly discovered that doctors and nurses belong to a closed society. They are extremely protective of their own. When word of the investigation got out, all doors seemed to close tighter than a bank vault.

However, I was successful in locating two witnesses who corroborated Bill MacKay's story in almost every respect. There were some inconsistencies, but these were minor in nature. Though reluctant, these witnesses were independent and totally credible. I now was confident that MacKay was telling the truth when he said that he participated in the surgery on Franklin Mirando. I now believed MacKay when he said he put together Mirando's fractured femur after it was splintered by David Lipton. I no longer doubted MacKay when he said that he reamed Mirando's femur and acetabulum. I was now forced to accept the fact that MacKay was truthful when he revealed that he inserted the prosthetic hip joint into the body of Franklin Mirando while the licensed medical people present observed and assisted him in silence.

At this point my investigation was almost complete, but there still remained one very difficult and painful thing to do. I had to confront the victim, Franklin Mirando, and inform him of my findings. Needless to say, I was nervous. At this point, I did not know if the July 1975 operation had been successful. I had never seen nor spoken to Mr. Mirando.

Sometime in late September, the inevitable meeting took place. My secretary informed me that Franklin Mirando and his wife were waiting to see me. I told her to show them into my office. She informed me that she could not do this, since the office would not be accessible to Mr. Mirando, who was in a wheelchair. When I heard this, I felt the blood drain from my face.

I arranged for a more convenient room and met with Franklin Mirando and his wife. At first I let them do the talking. Franklin told me about his disability. He advised me that he had been confined to a wheelchair since his "total hip" operation in July 1975. As a result of that operation, one leg is approximately two inches shorter than the other. He further advised that he had a malpractice suit pending against Dr. David Lipton because of a serious fracture to his femur during the course of the operation. From the tone of Mirando's conversation it was evident that he did not know anything about Bill MacKay.

When I finally told Franklin Mirando and his wife of the results of my investigation, they gasped and wept.

The Mirando case was submitted to a Suffolk County grand jury and an indictment returned against Drs. Lipton and Massoff, the anesthesiologist and Operating Room Supervisor Lorna Salzarullo, and the Smithtown General Hospital for assault in the second degree. In addition, Dr. Lipton and Nurse Salzarullo, along with the Smithtown General Hospital, were indicted under a separate indictment with Falsifying Business Records in the First Degree, also a felony.

After these indictments were handed down, a number of things occurred which, to my mind, carried political overtones and thrust the legislative and judicial systems into the controversy. Henry F. O'Brien, the Suffolk County District Attorney, under whose authority I conducted my investigation, was defeated in his bid for re-election. He was replaced by Patrick Henry, the current District Attorney, who days before the election stated that the Mirando case was a political issue. When Mr. Henry took office, all investigations into MacKay's past activities in Suffolk County were ordered stopped, and I was transferred to a non-investigative position. The defendants moved to dismiss the assault charges and their motion was granted. District Attorney Patrick Henry then moved to dismiss the remaining charges for Falsifying Business Records.

In this book, Mr. MacKay has opened the door and has shed substantial light on an appalling situation. But MacKay was one salesman, doing business in one particular geographic area. He sold specialized equipment to a limited number of surgeons. How many others are there who could relate experiences of equal or greater horror? Will we, the public, ever really know how far and wide the surgeon/salesman problem extends? As long as legislators and prosecutors treat the medical profession as a sacred cow, we will never know.

In conclusion, I would like to take this opportunity to thank Bill MacKay for opening my eyes. I also wish to thank him on behalf of the general public. Knowing at least some of the facts, patients may now begin to ask more questions and to obtain more answers from the medical profession. Thus, the public will be able to protect itself and to exert more pressure on elected officials to provide the legislation necessary for the public's safety.

ALBERT E. ARANEO

SALESMAN
SURGEON

ONE

THE FIRST TOTAL HIP

The surgeon studied the nine-by-five-inch patch of skin. It was painted a garish hue of orange and framed by green cotton sheets, a display of colors that meant the area was disinfected, draped, and ready to cut. Under the camouflage, the skin could have been an expanse of abdomen, back, or buttock. Actually, it was a right hip that a surgeon I will call Dr. Tom Merriman, Chief of Orthopedics at a hospital in Long Island, was about to lay open, saw, and replace with an artificial joint made of steel and plastic. He pondered where to make the incision, poking with his thumb for the greater trochanter, that protuberance of bone at the widest part of the hip. He touched not bare skin but Vidrape, a Saranlike plastic that encased the orange incision area as an added sterility precaution.

"Give me some methylene blue," Merriman ordered the scrub nurse. Martha O'Connell (I will call her) was standing at the foot of the operating table. She handed Merriman a special felt marking pen. Merriman, who sat on a stool facing the patient's right hip, drew a line to mark where he meant to cut. It began above the greater trochanter, curved downward in a 110-degree arc, then paralleled the outer side of the femur or thigh bone for about four inches. The entire line was about ten inches long, and blue. Soon it would turn red.

1

"Hand me the knife." Nurse O'Connell offered it with fingertips on the upper side of the blade, the plastic handle toward Merriman. She had seen many a scrub nurse's hand sliced by a surgeon who grabbed the scalpel too quickly. "Forceps," Merriman ordered. With scalpel in his right hand and forceps in his left, he began cutting the outer layer of skin, tracing the blue line downward from left to right, parting flesh and Vidrape in the same motion. A red line gradually widened in the wake. Merriman pinched the scalpel as a fastidious woman would a fine china teacup, between right thumb and index finger. He sliced an inch at a time, stopping, surveying his progress, moving steadily to the end of the line. He trailed the forceps just behind the scalpel, using it to separate the newly incised skin and give the knife space for the cutting that lay ahead.

I watched Merriman's hands from over his right shoulder. They were, like the rest of his body, slender but strong, much like the fine-boned, long-fingered hands most laymen expect of a surgeon. To Merriman's left was Dr. Arnold Kasik (again a pseudonym), the assistant surgeon. He was several years younger than Merriman and, at five feet eight inches, stood half a foot shorter. Kasik was an outgoing man with an affinity for good food and good company. Across the table stood Dr. Edward Janney, as I will name him. In street clothes, he looked younger than his fifty years. His hair was cropped close and his skin was tanned from a recent vacation in the Bahamas. Two orthopedic surgeons usually suffice for a total hip procedure, and I found myself wondering why Janney was there.

Merriman reached for a new scalpel and retraced the initial incision, cutting deeply this time, an inch into the fatty subcutaneous tissue known, in surgical hip talk, as the "subcue." He exchanged forceps for a sponge. With this large piece of gauze he dabbed at the blood on either side of his knife, for the incision was no longer merely leaking but was pumping a steady flow of blood. "Arnold, let's close off some of these bleeders." Merriman stopped cutting and clamped a forceps over a small capillary while Kasik touched the instrument with the pencillike wand of the Bovie electronic blood coagulator. A BZZZZZZ of electricity coursed through the metal forceps and burned the blood vessel permanently shut.

For the next five minutes, the two surgeons sealed off bleeders. Despite their efforts, blood was rapidly forming little pools inside the hip wound. Ever since Merriman had reached the subcue, Kasik had periodically dipped a thin tube into the incision to suction off blood and, using an instrument resembling a kitchen meat baster, had flooded the wound with antiseptic solution. This he also suctioned and sponged off. He handed the reddened sponges to the scrub nurse, who dropped them into a stainless-steel bucket on the floor. She would count them later to make sure none remained inside the patient.

Merriman had reached the hip capsule, a sack of tissue surrounding the joint itself. "Hand me the Bovie," he told Kasik. Merriman turned up the rheostat on the coagulating machine, surging enough power through the flat metal electrode tip not only to seal but to cut tissue. He began burning open the hip capsule. A stench suddenly filled the room. It was rancid, horrible, the aroma of dead flesh, and though I had smelled it before, I felt like leaving the room. The fumes curled in a vapor out of the hip cavity. Inside the hip capsule lay the part to be replaced, ordinarily the most mechanically perfect joint in the body but, in the case of the middle-aged man on the operating table, a hip devastated by arthritis.

As Merriman worked, the Bovie continued to BZZZZZZZZZ, BZZZZZZZZZZZZ, BZZZZZZZZZ, punctuating the usual routine chitchat that filled the room: "Gee, Dr. Kasik, you look like you've lost some weight."

"Yeah, I've been on a diet," Kasik said to Merriman. "I had to take my Cadillac in for service the other day. I've had it only three months, and already it's breaking down on me."

"I told you to get a Mercedes, Arnold. I love the things. Why don't you go to Tri-City Motors, where I bought mine? They'll give you a good deal."

"Nah, I don't feel like buying one of those German cars."

The small talk helped vent the excitement we all felt about this procedure. It was 1973 and total hip arthroplasty was big-league surgery, comparable in the orthopedic world to open-heart surgery in the cardiac. Earlier that morning, I had seen Merriman greeting the nurses with a wide smile and the lilt of anticipation in his voice as he moved down the hall: "Good morning." "Good morning." "Beautiful day." "How are you?" "How's everybody?" Behind his horn-rimmed glasses, his eyes sparkled. He had rubbed his hands together briskly as he strode toward the operating room, obviously looking forward to the procedure.

For nearly an hour Merriman's hands—and Kasik's—had been in perpetual motion, picking instruments up, setting them down. Merriman was ready to spread the incision with a U-shaped retractor that had rakelike attachments at the points of the U. Merriman cut another inch or two of skin so that Kasik could spread the incision about six inches wide. (Hip incisions tend to grow longer as a case progresses.)

Ordinarily the surgeon next removes the greater trochanter, the walnut-sized knob of bone Merriman had earlier felt with his thumb. This allows better access to the hip cavity. But in this case a problem intervened. The patient, during a previous operation, had had a device installed to repair a fracture at the top of the femur. Four bone screws held a plate to the thigh bone, and Merriman had to remove them all before cutting off the greater trochanter. The screws had, with age, become embedded in the bone, and Merriman had trouble removing them with a surgical screwdriver. After stripping the head of one screw, he finally turned it out with a vise grip.

The screw-removing interlude had bored Dr. Janney, judging from the way he was yawning under his mask and shifting from foot to foot. And the anesthesiologist, who had seemed oblivious to the drama of the initial incision, sat at the patient's head and read a book. I had seen this happen so often that I was not even curious to know the book's title.

I had been so absorbed in watching the operation that I had paid little attention to Dr. Janney. Suddenly I heard him announce, "Step 31 (Prepare to remove the femoral head)." This referred to the ball part of the ball-and-socket hip joint. Merriman responded by taking a Gigli saw, a flexible wire with teeth along its one-foot length, and snaking it around the neck of the femur with a forceps.

Suddenly I noticed that Janney was reading, too—from photo-copied instructions listing 120-odd steps for doing the Charnley total hip procedure, named for the doctor who invented the hip prosthesis we were installing. I had delivered the instructions to Merriman's office several days earlier, and now Janney was reading them aloud, one step at a time.

"Jesus Christ," I thought, "is he going to read _all_ 122 steps?"

As if in reply, Janney stretched across the patient's pelvis and peered inside the incision to see whether Merriman had finished Step 31.

"This is just like putting a kid's bicycle together on Christmas

Eve," I thought. "Don't these guys know what they're doing?" Never before had I seen instructions being read at a major—or even a minor—surgical procedure.

I began to comprehend the premeditation involved in bringing them into the operating room. The instructions, like everything else in the OR, needed to be sterilized. Obviously they could not be steamed in the autoclave along with the surgical instruments. The instruments had been sterilized instead with ethyl oxide gas, which requires at least two days to allow time for the residual gas fumes to disappear. This meant two days of advance planning, two days during which Merriman and Kasik could have committed the procedure to their heads rather than to paper. But written instructions were the method of choice—just like the checklist used by airline pilots. Janney's voice droned on.

"Step 33 (Cut the femoral neck)." Merriman began pulling the Gigli saw back and forth against the neck of the femur, his two hands moving like two men sawing a tree. He then took a flat chisel and completed his cut. Next he pried into the hip socket, struggling for about five minutes to break the suction seal between the femoral head and acetabulum, the socket of the hip joint. "Corkscrew," he told the scrub nurse, who handed him the appropriately named instrument. Merriman screwed it into the femoral head and pulled hard. At last the suction released. A piece of bone slightly larger than a golf ball popped out of the hip socket like a cork out of a bottle. Arthritis had distorted its natural shape and eroded its surface. Merriman dropped the bone into a stainless-steel specimen bowl which the scrub nurse set aside for the pathology laboratory.

Janney read off the next step and Merriman and Kasik moved the patient's leg into position for cutting a second slice off the femoral neck. They crossed the right leg over the left and pointed the right foot forward. Merriman then took a Gigli saw and cut the stump at a 40-to-50-degree angle. He judged it by eye because no instruments existed for measuring the angle. Yet if it is not precisely correct, the lower half of the hip prosthesis will not sit in the femoral canal properly and will not remain plugged into the hip socket later on.

"Step 50 (Ream the acetabulum)." The procedure had reached a critical phase. The way the hip socket is reamed determines how the plastic acetabular cup, which is the upper half of the body's new hip joint, will fit. Merriman began removing bone and cartilage from the hip socket and grinding its surface down to healthy, bleeding bone. He used a centering ring to mark the dead center of the acetabulum, where the bone should be thickest. Then, with a hand brace of the sort a carpenter uses to make holes in wood, he drilled completely through the acetabulum. This told him how thick it was so he would not remove too much bone. He turned the deepening reamer about two dozen times, excavating as far toward the center line of the body as possible. The better the center of gravity, the less the strain and the more stable the joint.

Merriman tried on the plastic acetabular cup for size, and drilled three holes the size of the tip of an index finger in the floor of the acetabulum. He worked carefully. Carelessly aimed, the drill could perforate the pelvis and injure major nerves, blood vessels, and other structures.

Janney began mixing bone cement, his other job, it turned out, besides reading the list of instructions. He dumped a white powder and liquid chemical into a stainless-steel bowl. With a sterilized spoon from the hospital cafeteria, he stirred just as a baker would mix eggs and flour. Janney worked quickly because the mixture, known as methylmethacrylate, sets in seven to eight minutes—sooner if the room is too warm. The other reason for haste is that bone cement produces horrible fumes, rivaling those of the hip capsule. Methylmethacrylate is an occupational hazard for nurses. They often develop headaches and eye irritation because they are exposed to the fumes far more than are the doctors. The cement quickly reached a doughlike consistency, and Janney removed it from the mixing bowl. He kneaded it between his thumbs and fingers as a baker might a piece of pastry and handed it to Merriman, who flattened it into a little pancake and pushed it with his fingers into the acetabulum.

Now came the tricky part: positioning the acetabular cup in the horizontal and vertical planes so that the leg would not dislocate. Merriman took a device used to position the acetabular cup and asked if I thought it was properly set. Up to this point, my role had been that of observer. I moved closer: "I believe it is."

"Should I antevert it a bit more?" he asked, meaning angle it upward toward the patient's navel.

"Why don't you give it just a touch," I said. Within minutes the cement hardened so that the cup could not be moved.

I glanced at the wall clock. It was 9:45 A.M. "Good," I said to

6

myself, "this is going to be a two-and-a-half-hour case with no complications."

Merriman was preparing to implant the femoral prosthesis. This is the lower half of the artificial hip joint. The lower end has a curved, pointed shaft and is cemented inside the medullary canal that runs down the center of the femur. At the upper end is a steel ball that fits into the acetabular cup. Merriman crossed the patient's right leg over the left and, with a rough file curved to the same shape as the femoral prosthesis, rasped the size hole necessary to accommodate it. Merriman tapped the instrument into the canal with a mallet, then banged it back out by striking a bar he inserted through its handle. Finished, he then drilled small holes through the femur so he could later rewire the greater trochanter, and inserted a trial femoral prosthesis without cementing it into place.

The patient was placed flat on his back for a trial reduction, a test of how the prosthesis fit. Kasik held his leg by the ankle and pulled until the prosthesis plugged into the acetabular cup. When he released the leg, the hip muscles worked as rubber bands and held the joint together. Merriman and Kasik moved the patient's leg in all directions and made sure both legs were the same length. They also checked the angle of the femoral prosthesis, for here—as in the acetabulum—the wrong angle could cause the leg to dislocate. Yet no instrument exists for positioning the prosthesis. It is done by eye. The leg seemed perfect, although a trial reduction does not prove much because the uncemented femoral prosthesis is apt to be loose and wobbly. Merriman withdrew the prosthesis and Dr. Janney began mixing a second batch of methylmethacrylate cement. He handed it to Merriman, who rolled it into a cigar shape and pushed it, between thumb and little finger, into the hollowed-out shaft of the femur. Merriman embedded the femoral prosthesis into the cement, which soon became rock-hard.

A few minutes later, Dr. Kasik pulled the leg by the ankle again to plug the femoral component into the artificial hip socket. But as soon as Kasik released the leg, the right foot and knee flopped toward the right. A look of dismay crossed Merriman's face. This meant the worst kind of trouble: the prosthesis had fallen out of the acetabular cup and the leg had dislocated. He rummaged inside the hip and said, "Let's try it again." Kasik again pulled on the leg, but as soon as he let go, it flopped to the right. Something was wrong, and everybody knew it. Apparently

Merriman had placed the femoral prosthesis in at the wrong angle, possibly because of the way he cut the femoral neck earlier in the procedure, possibly because there was no instrument to help him position the prosthesis. Merriman had not asked my opinion about its positioning because he had been installing a similar type of femoral device for years. It was an honest error that stemmed not from carelessness or incompetence but a genuine, if mistaken, belief that he had done the right thing.

The immediate problem was not why the error had occurred but what to do next. And nobody, including me, knew the answer to that question.

Panic began to invade the room. It affected Merriman worst of all. Perspiration started to roll down his face, and I could see in his expression the growing realization that the prosthesis would have to be removed and inserted all over again. One could almost see the thought of a malpractice suit flashing through his mind.

"Jesus, what did I do wrong?" he said. "What do I do now?"

Janney was stuttering: "M-m-maybe it will be okay when we rewire the greater trochanter." He was referring to the bone removed earlier to give the surgeons more operating room.

Merriman pulled down the trochanter, hoping the muscles attached to it created enough tension to hold the femoral component in the cup. It didn't work.

Fifteen minutes had elapsed since disaster struck. Suddenly Merriman turned to me: "I'll tell you what we are going to do," he said. "We are going to make an incision at the distal end of the femur, just above the knee, and I will take a saw and cut directly through the entire femur and turn the femur in my hand to put it in the right degree of anteversion. Then we will take an Elliot femoral condyle plate and screw the bone back together." In plain English, Merriman wanted to saw the largest bone in the body—the femur—in half just above the knee and turn it to compensate for a misalignment of the prosthesis in the hip area! Then he proposed to reattach the two pieces of femur with a steel bone plate and screws. He already had an eight-inch incision in the hip, and now he wanted to cut the same leg at the knee!

Janney and I looked at each other in amazement. Then we turned toward Merriman and told him that there was no way on earth he could do this.

I added that his idea probably would not work anyway. Worse, it would expose the patient to additional infection, trauma, and bleeding. I had never heard of any case where sawing the femur in half was a solution for anything—unless it was an amputation.

After a long silence, Merriman looked at me. "Okay, what should I do?"

"The first thing you do, Doctor," I replied, "is take out the femoral prosthesis."

Merriman took a mallet and started tapping the femoral component, trying to knock it toward the patient's head. His strokes were dainty and getting nowhere.

"Hit it harder," I said.

Tap, tap, tap, tap, tap, tap. Still nothing happened.

He gave me a pained look and said, "Here, you do it."

I took the mallet and landed one strong blow under the head of the prosthesis. It flew out of the patient's femur and hit the wall ten feet across the room with a bang. But at least it was out of the patient. I began to have a feeling of relief. I had never seen the revision of a prosthesis before. I had read about it, I had heard about it. But I had never practiced it or seen the procedure performed.

As I peered at the cement still inside the femoral canal, Merriman said, "How do we get that out of there?" I suggested using osteotomes (bone chisels). Merriman took one and started chipping away at the cement, but again he showed little progress or perseverance. After two more minutes of chipping, he lost his temper and yelled at me, "Bill, get over here and take out this fucking cement! This is ridiculous."

Suddenly Dr. Janney announced that he had to go conduct office hours. We hardly noticed him leave.

To remove the cement we had to fragment it, so I suggested using medullary reamers, which are oversized drills much like those the telephone-company installer uses when he runs a phone line through a wall. It occurred to me that this drill, with its two-inch cutting tip, might be even more effective with a power source. Dr. Merriman asked the operating-room supervisor for the medullary reamers and an orthotome drill, which operates at 750 rpm. She returned with them and hooked the drill air hose to the nitrogen tank at the side of the room. Merriman tackled the cement again.

Nothing happened.

"Just keep reaming," I said. I could see his frustration mounting because he could not get the cement out.

"Come over here and show me how to do it," he said.

I stood in Merriman's place and went to work on the femur. But the drill was jumping around and bouncing off the cement. I decided to honeycomb the cement with a bit like that on a regular household drill. After weakening the cement, I returned to the medullary reamer. Finally, as I was leaning on it, the cement started to yield.

Merriman was giving oral aid in the meantime, offering such comments as "You're doing a great job," "That's terrific," "Keep going."

I occasionally stopped drilling and chipped at the cement with an osteotome to break it down further. The cement fragments ranged in size from half a matchstick to a pencil eraser. The larger pieces I removed with a forceps until the canal was clean. Only then did I realize that I had been working on the cement one hour and a half. It seemed as if time had stood still. I told Merriman he could insert the new femoral component. "You are doing okay," he said. "You put it in." Kasik began mixing another smelly batch of methylmethacrylate. I worked it down the shaft, then inserted the prosthesis, carefully checking the angle.

When the cement set, Kasik pulled down the patient's right leg and plugged the prosthesis into the acetabular cup, hopefully for the last time. The fit was perfect. I felt a surge of satisfaction and relief as Merriman and I wired the greater trochanter back in place. Merriman closed the remaining layers of tissue, leaving a suction tube to drain blood from deep inside the wound. He placed an abduction pillow between the patient's legs to keep him from moving around and dislocating the hip. A technician took two postoperative X rays, a front and a side view, and an orderly wheeled the patient into the recovery room.

An operation that normally should have taken about three hours had stretched on for six. As we were leaving the operating room, the OR supervisor said, "I'm glad that's over," and Dr. Merriman thanked me for helping out. "We can really use a guy like you," he said.

With that, he and Kasik walked down the hall to make their rounds, and I left to make mine. I was going to call on another hospital, but not to see patients. I was not an orthopedic surgeon; I had never been to medical school. I was a medical-supply salesman.

TWO
ME SALESMAN

My "medical" career began in 1973 when on a sunny August day I was handed an orthopedic equipment catalog. It listed about 5500 items, most of which I had never heard of before. The catalog included just about everything man (or, to put it more precisely, the biomechanical engineers at my company's laboratories) could devise for repairing human bones and joints. When I first thumbed through it, I thought I must be working for the world's largest hardware store. The stock included staples, bands, nails, clips, screws, clamps, wires, awls, rasps, chisels, drills, gouges, mallets, and saws. Half a dozen artificial total hips were listed, each in a range of sizes. There were illustrations of instruments with unpronounceable names: intertrochanteric plates, osteotomes, rongeurs. There were Jewett nails, Parham bands, Steinmann pins, Kuntscher intramedullary nails, Hall II air drivers—and more. In time I would have to learn every item in this imposing catalog. But for now I was to sell only one, a special hospital mattress designed to prevent bedsores. My boss, whom I will call Harry Fontaine, never trusted new salesmen with the entire line. As usual, he decided to test me out on mattresses. I was starting from scratch. But I had done it before.

11

My working career began when I was thirteen, when I was suspended from Garden City High School on Long Island after completing the first four days of ninth grade. In truth, I wanted to be thrown out. I had attended a series of military schools during grade school. But I did not enjoy marching to other people's drums.

I had always had skill using my hands. During childhood they had fashioned airplane models, dollhouses, a music box for my mother. But at age thirteen horses were my real love. I wanted to become a professional show rider and get rich, of course, in the process. For five years I worked for horse trainers in Virginia, Kentucky, Pennsylvania, Michigan, and New York. I did not get rich.

At seventeen I was hurt badly when the gelding I was riding went *into* instead of *over* a jump, flipped in midair, and 1400 pounds of horseflesh landed on me. I broke more bones than I care to remember, and spent weeks in the hospital. When I recovered, my doctor told me that I would be unwise to ride again.

I needed a job—any kind of job—and found one as a dishwasher at the Hamburger Express in Garden City, Long Island. I had no other skills and washing greasy plates was quite a setback after running with the horsey set. Fortunately, the hamburger break was brief.

My next employer was a tree surgeon. One day we were in Seacliff, Long Island, doctoring one of the splendid old trees that grace the community. We were hanging way up in the air, with only a rope and a sling to preserve us, when suddenly my rope broke and I plummeted to the ground. By some miracle, only the wind was knocked out of me. I looked up and saw my boss, still dangling from his rope amid the foliage. "Are you hurt?" he shouted.

"No, I'm all right."

"Well, come on back."

I looked up, said "Fuck you," and walked away. I never went back.

My next job was in auto body work, banging out bent fenders, a job that caused blisters and sore muscles. After about six months, I knew I did not want to earn my living that way. Then, one day I walked into an employment agency in Hempstead, Long Island, and told the man I was looking for a job.

He said, "Why not work here?"

"As what?" I asked.

"As a counselor."

"I don't even own a suit," I said.

"Go buy one," he replied.

That was in 1965. I worked there until 1967, when I decided to open my own agency.

My partner and I opened our agency in December 1969, with fifteen hundred dollars between us, some rented folding chairs, and an aluminum picnic table. The place was previously a doctor's office. When we moved in, it looked like an old bus station, only not as good. But we worked long hours, earned enough to redecorate three months later, and within twelve months sold thirteen franchises in five states, including New York. Toward the end of 1970, I began to feel that franchising in general was headed downhill, and I sold my share of the partnership in January 1971. I then opened William MacKay Associates, an executive recruitment firm in Garden City, Long Island. The business thrived until July 1973 when, after one of my customary eighteen holes of golf in the rain, I contracted pneumonia. It developed into pleurisy and I was hospitalized for about a month. I returned to find my business in sad neglect. When two of my employees offered to buy the firm, I accepted.

During employment-business days, I had met Harry Fontaine when he had come to me looking for employees. He asked me if I would like to sell medical equipment. At the time I was interested, but not enough to switch businesses. Now, in the late summer of 1973, I wanted the job badly. For one thing, the money that orthopedic-equipment salesmen earn was enticing. I sensed a chance to work hand-in-hand with doctors. Before I had fallen in love with horses, the foremost fantasy of my childhood was to become an MD. I also craved the continuity of clients who would come back and reorder a product, rather than disappear after I found them a job. The security of a big corporation also attracted me. After so many years of maverick existence, I was ready for a change. I called Harry and we met. A week later he called and offered me a job. The next afternoon at the King's Grant Motel in Plainview, he handed me the company's catalog and told me to start reading.

As I turned the pages that night, looking at the artificial implants, the surgical instruments, the hospital equipment and supplies, I came to a section at the back titled "Surgical Techniques." It contained step-by-step descriptions of various medical procedures for replacing hips and knees, for pinning and mending hips, and for inserting rods into the body to straighten spines deformed by scoliosis. The introduction noted that this section had been included as an "educational aid" for the surgeon and his paramedical staff. But even at that early stage, I sensed another motive.

The events those pages foreshadowed were still in the future. My immediate concern was with the mattress Harry gave me to sell. The catalog heralded it as the solution to the decubitus ulcer problem. This mattress, in other words, supposedly prevented bedsores, which are caused by the pressures of lying on the same part of the body—especially the bony parts—for long periods of time. I started making rounds of hospitals convincing the nurses to order several on trial. When the mattresses arrived, I would return to the hospital and give the nursing personnel an "in-service" (orientation) program to show them how the mattresses worked and why they were so special. The nurses became so eager to check the mattresses out that they turned the patients frequently. As a result, the patients could have been lying on concrete and, with that kind of nursing care, would not have developed bedsores!

Two weeks later, with the patients still "clean"—free of bedsores—the nurses would tell me: "Mr. MacKay, these mattresses are *fantastic!*" At that point I would strike home and sell one for every bed in the hospital, even though it was triple the price of the mattress it replaced. Hospitals, for inventory purposes, buy such items en masse, placing the order for a 200-bed institution at about $24,000. All things considered, price above all, the antiulcer mattress was probably one of the greatest razzle-dazzle schemes on the market.

I sold so many of these mattresses that about three months later I was called to Harry Fontaine's office and told I could handle the entire line of equipment. Harry also gave me twenty hospital accounts. They were the worst hospitals in the worst areas of his entire territory, hospitals doing little or no business with my company, hospitals in Brooklyn and Queens where I walked in the door and hoped to leave in one piece.

One day I visited a hospital in Brooklyn to show an operating-room supervisor a dermatome, a skin-grafting device. I could see that she had no intention of buying it. She was merely going through the motions so she could tell the doctor who had requested the instrument that she had priced it and found it too expensive. Following this familiar and fruitless ritual, I returned to my station wagon in the back lot of the hospital. In the distance I spotted half a dozen teen-age boys perched on the hood of my car and leaning against it. Normally, I would have retreated to the hospital and returned in twenty minutes, hoping they would be gone. But on this day I had an appointment, so I braced myself and walked straight toward my car, door key in hand. I decided not to put my equipment bag in the rear end and invite twelve hands to pilfer back there. As I reached the car I said, "Hi, guys, how're you doing?" got in, locked the door, and immediately started the motor. To my relief, several punks jumped off the hood. But two remained looking angrily at me even after I raced the motor for a moment, and I smelled trouble. So I gunned the motor and drove off, swerving to slide off the two as I raced across the parking lot. Had I hesitated, I am sure they would have done more than sit on my car. When at last I reached the street, my pounding heart told me how frightened I was.

One Bronx hospital, also on my calling list, was a veritable war zone: even doctors had been knifed in this hospital. One day another salesman led me to a door to peer through a small glass window into a large auditorium once used for teaching. I saw perhaps a hundred men and women dressed in the jackets and dungarees that gang members wear. Immediately two tough-looking young men opened the swinging door and asked, "Can we help you?" The words were polite, but the real message was menacing. I told them I was a medical-equipment salesman and was looking around the hospital. "Well," one said, "this is a private meeting room. You'd better go about your business." I did. My salesman friend explained that the hospital had turned the auditorium over to a gang which terrorized the South Bronx. "If any other toughs come walking by," he advised, "just keep smiling."

Again, in the emergency room of another hospital in the Bronx, I saw a young boy brought in with a chest wound. I watched the staff scurry about, putting tubes down his throat and helping him breathe, because he was drowning in his own blood. Suddenly about eight gang members appeared in the doorway in full fighting regalia. They carried chains in their hands. One held a rifle, another stood glowering with a knife big enough to decapitate a cow with one swipe. They were after the boy with the chest wound. The only thing that kept them from killing him was a New York City policeman brandishing a gun.

I once told a friend after a hoodlum tried to mug me in a hospital: "I fight for my life at least once a month in this city." Those first few months while Harry Fontaine was testing me were really tough. He reasoned that if I could sell the worst hospitals—and I did—I could certainly sell in the good ones. About eight months later, another salesman left and I was given twenty-one accounts in the Nassau-Suffolk territory on Long Island. The area was a plum.

During my mattress-selling days, I had noticed that there are two kinds of salesmen: those who take orders and run errands for doctors, and those who know their equipment and demonstrate it to surgeons in the operating room. I decided to become the latter kind because, among other things, they make the most money. I also decided to become the best medical-equipment salesman in the business. This meant, for starters, knowing the equipment, which I could not do merely by reading catalogs. Harry Fontaine was a great help in this respect. He would sit at my dining-room table on a Saturday or Sunday morning, spread out the various artificial joints or implants, and teach me how each one is used. After fifteen years in the business he had become an expert on metallurgy and internal fixation, the medical term for repairing and replacing damaged bones and joints. He not only helped me sell the equipment, he taught me more about implants than most doctors learn in any medical school or hospital residency program.

The unfamiliarity of the average surgeon regarding artificial joints is chronic. Ever since 1960, when artificial hip joints were in their infancy, Dr. John Charnley (the real name of the British orthopedic surgeon who developed the Charnley total hip prosthesis) has stressed that the implantation of artificial hips demands training in mechanical techniques that are not taught during the education of a surgeon. Yet these techniques are elementary to the student of practical engineering. Charnley has recommended establishing centers to teach reconstructive surgery of the hip joint, preferably in league with the engineering departments of local universities. These centers, he notes, could train surgeons in a variety of techniques and make them more than one-operation men.

In my own specialty, selling orthopedic equipment, I had no intention of becoming a one-operation man. I became fascinated by the variety of artificial hips, knees, ankles, and the intricacies of implanting them in the human body. Soft goods such as slings and braces seemed dull by comparison, and I found myself spending two-thirds of my day selling implants, not by reading the catalog to doctors but by telling them what I thought they needed. I would take with me when I called on a doctor a new total hip prosthesis, for example, and show him how my product worked better than the one he was currently using and how it could bring the patient to weight-bearing capacity more quickly. The bottom line, of course, was that the company, the doctor, and I were all looking to put the patient back on his feet as fast as possible.

My selling job was aided by constant changes in the products themselves. Some of the most advanced devices available today may be obsolete within five years. While I sold orthopedic equipment, at least ten different total hips crowded the market. Artificial hips were just coming into their own during the early 1970s, and three or four major design changes and at least thirty minor modifications took place. They changed from metal on metal to metal on plastic, to no-stem, to different-length stems, to modifications in the necks, to modifications in the cup. Not all the changes were improvements. When I entered the orthopedic-equipment business, the hip in vogue was implanted with no cement by driving spikes into the acetabulum. To install one prosthesis, the surgeon screwed the acetabular cup into the pelvis. The trouble is that anything that is screwed in can screw out, and that is exactly what happened. One doctor designed a hip that featured, in the femoral head, a bearing larger than a large marble. After three or four months, the bearing wore down so badly that the entire device had to be replaced. This meant more surgery for the patient. Another hip, of Russian design, was installed by pounding the cup into the acetabulum with a hammer. Sometimes, while the surgeon pounded it in, the cup became brown with feces because it kept going right through the pelvis.

The changes also created problems for the doctors. They were confronted with a bewildering array of implants to choose from. Every time an implant changed, so did the surgical technique. Installing total hip A differed from installing total hip B, making it difficult for doctors to keep abreast of technology. Thus they increasingly came to rely upon the technical expertise of representatives from the various medical-equipment companies.

Beside knowing the implants, being the best salesman also

meant outdoing the competition. Eight other orthopedic companies employed about forty salesmen in the New York City area, and each sold essentially the same devices. The total hip invented by Dr. John Charnley was, for example, manufactured and sold by three different companies. The Müller hip was also sold by three competing companies. It was extremely difficult to patent a medical device because a company could make a slight modification and call it a Charnley-type total hip. At an average cost of about $350 per hip and a commission of nine percent, the competition to sell was fierce.

Competitive practices in selling medical equipment, like those in other fields, ranged from the primitive to the sophisticated. At the primitive level, salesmen would lie about one another professionally and personally. One, for example, might enter a hospital and learn that his competitor had, the day before, told the staff he gives poor service or that the product he sells has had many clinical failures. Or a salesman might tell a doctor, "Did you hear that So-and-So really screwed up at Blank-Blank hospital?" His competitors might retaliate: "Did you know ____ Company just had a price increase?" when, in fact, it had not.

A salesman attempting to discredit a competitor's character might tell a happily married operating-room supervisor that his colleague was about to leave his wife and family for another woman. When I divorced and remarried in October 1975, some people claimed, "My God, he stole the operating-room supervisor at Hospital X away from a doctor." Competition at its worst led one salesman to pour five pounds of Domino sugar down another's gas tank. One day I walked out of a hospital and found all four tires slashed.

Even within the company, the salesmen vied against one another. We all wanted to be Harry Fontaine's Number One Boy. The salesman in New York would come into the office and claim "Dr. So-and-So is complaining about the Queens salesman." My favorite competitive ploy was to give spectacular sales presentations, complete with charts and graphs, at Harry's monthly meetings. My performances helped win me the general sales manager's position for the New York area.

At the most rewarding level, a good salesman knew his products better than any of his competitors. For example, two salesmen might sell essentially the same air drill, at the same price, at exhibit tables in the same room of the same hospital. The question, then, becomes: Does Salesman A know more about his equipment than Salesman B knows about his? Can Salesman A impart that knowledge to the doctor and convince him he knows more? Can Salesman A build rapport with that doctor? If Salesman A ever gets caught not knowing what he is talking about, the doctor will lose faith in him. But if Salesman A gains the doctor's confidence, a closer relationship will develop. The salesman will learn the doctor's capabilities (or lack of them) and the two will begin, basically, to communicate.

The doctor wants somebody in whom he can place confidence. He does not want to summon five salesmen and evaluate five knees to decide which is best. He does not want to read a ten-page brochure. What he does want is to tell (hopefully) Bill MacKay: "I'm doing a total knee a week from today," and then forget about it, because he knows that I will have the knee and all the instruments he needs in the operating room that day. More important, he knows I will be there in case of problems with the equipment or, as I recounted earlier, with the case itself. The knee I sell may be the best in the world, or the worst, but the reason the doctor buys that prosthesis is because I sell it.

Another complexity is that medical equipment must be sold not only to doctors but also to the hospital personnel—especially the supply and operating-room people. An operating-room supervisor can decide which hip or knee prosthesis will be used regardless of what the doctor wants. She can exercise this kind of power because she controls other things the doctor needs. For example, the doctor wants to start surgery at 7 A.M. or 8 A.M. so he can hold early-afternoon office hours. But the supervisor sets the operating-room schedule. If he gives her any grief, he will find himself in surgery at 11 A.M. instead of 8, and he will be late for 1 P.M. office hours. The surgeon may ask the OR supervisor to order a certain total hip through the purchasing department and she may reply, "I'm sorry, doctor, we don't use those hips in this hospital. You'll have to use what we have." Medical-equipment salesmen will find themselves in the middle in this type of situation. We have to sell to the doctor *and* the OR personnel.

The latter are not easily sold. For one thing, OR supervisors are busy people, even busier than doctors in some instances. They have an operating room to run, with intricate schedules to meet, nurses to handle, doctors to appease. These OR people are not asking to be sold anything. In fact, they are trying to shoot down the salesman with arguments that his equipment is not compatible with the equipment already in the hospital. When this happens, the salesman must convince the supervisor that Company X's equipment is better and that he can make it compatible. The OR supervisor might object that she would have to buy new instruments to install Company X's particular prosthesis. The astute salesman then offers a starter set of surgical instruments. For a total hip procedure these cost $5000 to $6000 retail, but do not cost the hospital a dime. Nobody loses because the hospital starts buying its total hips (and, in time, most of its other equipment) from Company X.

Ultimately, the salesman sells hospital personnel the same thing as he sells the doctors: service. So when an OR supervisor would ask me to deliver an out-of-stock item, I would jump in my car and deliver it immediately, just as I would for a doctor.

I worked for Harry Fontaine until October 1975, when I became the Long Island distributor for a competing orthopedic equipment company. I had just remarried, and my wife and I started the business on a metal table in our apartment. My new employer had been doing little business in the New York area, and we spent 1976 building a sales force and rapport with the hospitals. By the year's end we had a healthy business that generated good income and employed five salesmen plus a secretary.

On a typical day I would leave the house at seven in the morning. Harry Fontaine had trained me to arrive at my first hospital by eight, and I never lost the habit. I would go straight to the operating room with two dozen doughnuts under my arm for the nurses to have with their coffee. It was an unwritten law that any salesman who failed to bring doughnuts for the girls was a son-of-a-bitch.

Then I would talk to the OR supervisor for a few minutes, go to the emergency room to speak to the ER supervisor about an equipment order, then to central supply to see about a new product. Next I would visit some doctors in the hospital. During the next few hours, I might end up in surgery, make sales rounds of another hospital, visit a clinic, or give an in-service training program to teach the nursing personnel how to apply knee braces. I might visit a hospital administrator to discuss the purchase of $25,000 to $30,000 worth of traction equipment, which represents a major capital expenditure, or meet with the head of a purchasing department about a new contract for the forthcoming year. Around 3 P.M. I would stop working in hospitals and do nothing but call on doctors in their offices. At one stop, I might show the doctor some new products, at another he might show me X rays of a patient about to receive a total knee or hip.

Once I showed a doctor a new ankle my company had just designed. He immediately called his secretary for X rays of Patient X, and decided to implant the device because this patient was "a beautiful candidate." The doctor had planned to fuse the ankle—to "weld" the joint surgically with small chips of bone from adjoining areas. This would make the ankle pain-free but no longer movable, which hardly mattered since the joint was already arthritic and had very little motion. Many doctors, I found, were willing to do a total ankle, total knee, or whatever because I dropped it in their laps. Occasionally I would visit a doctor to look at X rays of a patient who needed a total hip. I would set a template over the film and show the doctor which of the several hips I sold might be suitable for that patient.

My official day as a salesman would end around five or six o'clock, but not my working day. Weekends, for example, were often preempted by doctors calling to borrow projectors and films on surgical techniques. A doctor once called me at ten one Sunday morning because the bulb for the projector I loaned him had burned out.

"What about the spare bulb?" I asked.

"I don't know how to put it in!" he replied. So I left my family and the Sunday *New York Times* and drove half an hour to his house to replace a burned-out bulb.

No sooner had I returned to the Sunday paper than the doctor called back: "Hey, the light bulb blew and I need another one!" (Not "Where can I buy another bulb?" but "I *need* another one.") This kind of thoughtlessness was commonplace.

One day I was at another hospital that had just agreed to loan a hospital fifteen miles distant some special diagnostic lights, which are used in pediatric wards. These lights are large and cumbersome, yet the hospital staff thought nothing of asking me to transport them across town. Had I refused, the next time these people ordered equipment, it would not have been from me.

On another occasion, a hospital in Queens needed a special traction apparatus to fit on the wheelchair of a patient with scoliosis, a serious curvature of the spine. This hospital had a maintenance department, carpenters, metal workers, and many others equipped to build mechanical devices. But they asked me to make the wheelchair frame for them, and expected it free of charge.

Time and again, a doctor would book a case two weeks in advance. But the OR supervisor, for one reason or another, would fail to order the prosthesis or borrow the instruments. On the morning of the procedure, while the patient was lying on a stretcher outside the OR, somebody would call me in panic: "Where are the instruments? Where is the implant?"

"You didn't order them," I would say.

"Well, we need them _right away_. Can you get them here in an hour?"

One doctor who wanted to do a total knee summoned me to his house after he finished evening office hours. When I arrived at the appointed time, his wife announced that he was performing surgery because it was the only time he could reserve the OR. I drove to the hospital and showed him a movie of the total knee procedure at midnight. At seven the next morning I delivered the prosthesis to the hospital where he was doing surgery, only to be told that the operation had been canceled.

Salesmen were also expected, as part of their unofficial duties, to convince their companies to manufacture the pet projects of various doctors. One, for example, devised a special heel for a cast boot that, in my opinion, would have overextended the patient's ankle and cause him to lose motion in that joint. After I rejected his invention, the doctor took it to a competitor, who agreed to form an orthopedic soft goods company and market the cast-boot heel. The other salesman went along with the scheme because he was trying to wean the doctor's business away from me. But he had no illusions about the cast-boot heel. At one point he joked with me about it in the lobby of a hospital.

Another surgeon invented a hip prosthesis that he had tried for years to sell to an orthopedic company. I helped persuade my company to manufacture this product, and as soon as the royalty agreement was signed, I received a $10,000 traction-equipment order, plus other orders that I had never received before. All told, my business at his hospital increased from $1000 to more than $20,000 a year. It was the doctor's way of saying thank you.

Still, a salesman's best business depended upon his ability to offer service, technical advice, and more, during surgery. Any salesman who fails to provide these amenities is in deep trouble. If a surgeon asks a salesman to scrub in on a case and is declined, he will ask a competitor instead and he will buy from that competitor thereafter. Willingness to attend surgery is the key, and once a salesman enters the OR, he can hardly refuse to hand the surgeon an instrument, or hold a retractor, or. . . .

When I first realized that this was how the medical-equipment business worked, I was both horrified and fascinated. I was upset by the reward-for-favor basis of the medical-equipment business, by the errand-running I saw other salesmen doing, and the errands I ran myself. I was repelled by having to tolerate many other detestable practices I will describe in this book. At the same time, I enjoyed the satisfactions of successfully building up a clientele, of working for a challenging boss, and of matching wits on a daily basis with competitors. I liked the excitement of the medical profession and—at the outset, at least—the godlike aura of doctors. I was attracted by the deep involvement with the orthopedic community that my job entailed and by the feeling, for the first time in my life, that I belonged to something. Above all, however, I was fascinated by the lure of the operating room.

Harry Fontaine had hinted at my surgical future the day he hired me: "This is not a job for the squeamish, Bill. You're going to be helping doctors. You're going to see people in the emergency room, the operating room. You're going to see blood, and you have to be prepared for that." And I had said, "Right!" I was fully prepared. Harry never told me to scrub in or participate in surgery, but I felt that the inference was there. It was a matter of individual interpretation and I knew what conclusion I—and many of my colleagues—were expected to reach.

Two years later, in 1974, Harry asked me to sign a letter saying I would not participate or scrub in on any surgery in hospitals in my territory. But he handed me the paper in a tongue-in-cheek way that said he needed it for legal cover. He said, "I'm telling you officially not to do surgery. If you do, it will blow up in your face someday." I did not believe him. I felt that he had lost touch with the profession. He was not out making sales, and it was easy to cite the rulebook. I also felt that because he, and not the company, employed me, he probably also feared personal liability.

Company directives might have been murky, but from other quarters the expectations were clear. The day before the total hip case I described earlier, after I had delivered the instruments and oriented the operating-room staff—which, like me, had never done the Charnley total hip procedure before—the scrub nurse said, "I'd like you to be here tomorrow." The operating-room supervisor was more direct: "Our last salesman was *always* here when we wanted him. I expect you here tomorrow morning at seven-thirty sharp!"

I went home that night and reread the Charnley procedure in textbooks and journals I had collected.

The next morning I arrived at the hospital at the appointed hour, went to the operating room, entered the doctor's lounge, and put on greens.

THREE

MAKING OF
A SURGEON

Some surgeons go to Stanford or Harvard. The rest attend one of about 120 other medical schools scattered across the country. Then they spend another four years or so learning their specialty. My medical education took place in the garage behind my house in Stony Brook, Long Island, in hospital emergency rooms, surgical suites, cafeterias, corridors, morgues, and autopsy rooms. When I began selling medical equipment, it became obvious that success in the business would require a tremendous amount of self-education. If a doctor said he had to trim a condyle or position the acetabular cup, I had to know what he meant so that, hopefully, I could sell him an instrument for doing it better. My aim was to become a good salesman, not a surgeon. In the process, I discovered that the best teachers I had were the doctors themselves.

One surgeon in particular was my mentor. He was the Chief of Orthopedics at a major teaching hospital in Queens, and I will call him Dr. Bruce Agee because, like many other doctors in this book, I do not wish to identify him. I met him several days after receiving my first twenty accounts in 1973, and told him I was new in the business and eager to learn. Dr. Agee must have sensed my interest, because he invited me to attend conferences and work with his orthopedic residents, even though he could have gotten into deep trouble for allowing this. He did not need to ask twice. Although he did not specifically invite me into the emergency room, I showed up several evenings later and put on a white lab coat. When Dr. Agee walked in and saw me there with the other residents, he gave me a little smile and said, "Oh, hi, Bill." I think he was surprised to see me, but pleased that I had taken the time and interest to be there. Within four hours I was making ward rounds with the residents.

At first I just watched. There was plenty to see. Several nights after I started, the police brought in a man around midnight. He arrived in a police car because there was no time to wait for an ambulance, for his stomach was ripped open and part of his intestines were hanging out. We were transferring him to surgery when a woman rushed into the emergency room, screaming and crying, "Oh, my God, where is he? My husband, my husband!"

"How did this happen?" the resident asked her.

"I cut him good. Next time I catch him fucking around I'll cut his throat!"

Two minutes earlier she had been crying, "Oh, my poor husband." But when she remembered why she had stabbed him, she wanted to finish the job, and the police had to restrain her. Anyway, her wayward husband was taken to surgery, where the residents sewed him up without further complication, at least from the medical standpoint.

Another time I walked into the emergency room to discover a policeman standing with his hand on his holster, guarding a wounded prisoner. The man had been shot three times, and he was lying on a stretcher outside the operating room, unconscious and bleeding heavily.

"What are you guarding him for?" I asked the officer. "He's not going anywhere."

"I'm guarding him all the way!"

"There's no way in the world that he's going to get up," I insisted.

In fact, the man died in the operating room. He had three bullet holes in him, and this enforcer of the law was looking to put in number four.

The only reason the orthopedic residents were involved with the patient with three gunshot wounds was that two bullets had shattered his left shoulder. While taking care of those, the residents did not realize that a third bullet had lodged at the base of the heart. That was the one that killed him. More typical of our everyday caseload was the kid who fell off the fire escape and broke his leg or the elderly woman who walked out to empty the garbage pail, slipped on the ice, and broke her hip.

On weekends something happened every minute. We would send for a pizza from the neighborhood parlor, and no sooner would it arrive than an emergency would arrive, too, and the pizza would sit there and get cold. We had accidents, suicides, stabbings, gunshot wounds. Victims of a two-car wreck would come in, three from one car, four from the other, all broken and bleeding so badly that we could not tell what color they were. A known prostitute would say she had been raped. People would come in with the tops of their heads hanging off, their arms broken, their teeth knocked out, their noses broken. This place was, as one of the residents described it, like being in Vietnam.

For three months I sold mattresses by day and worked in the emergency room by night. I arrived around 5 P.M., stayed until eleven or twelve o'clock, got to bed around one, and was up and running at six. On Friday nights I usually stayed all night, and sometimes on weeknights as well. Saturday I stayed home with my family but, by Sunday, I was back on the wards. At first my role was watching or holding an arm while the residents patched it up. By the third week I was cutting sutures for the residents and by week four I was doing some suturing. A resident supervised: "Make your knots tighter." "Make your knots closer." "The more stitches you have, the less noticeable the scar on this part of the body."

The man who taught me most about this art was a salesman from one of the leading manufacturers of sutures. He had never touched a patient, but he was very handy at suturing. One day, over lunch in a pancake restaurant, he showed me how to set up a suture on a needleholder. This device, which resembles a scissors with a gripping end, grasps the needle while the surgeon wraps the suture or surgical thread around it. When the half-moon-shaped needle pierces the skin, the person doing the suturing releases the holder, reaches for the tip of the needle, and pulls it through. The suture emerges ready for tying the knot that draws the pieces of skin together. Then the surgeon (or whoever) takes the suture in his left hand, holds the end of the needle in his right, ties a knot, and cuts the thread. Moving up

27

the incision, he repeats the process. I sat in the pancake house and practiced on the crust of a piece of toast while he kept telling me what a klutz I was. Then he gave me several boxes of sutures to take home, where I tried various stitches on a piece of fabric. After a week or so, I became proficient at suturing.

During this period Dr. Agee started treating me more and more like one of his residents. I attended orthopedic conferences and lectures, taking an hour or two from sales rounds during the day, and Dr. Agee asked me questions just as he would the residents. Whenever an X ray involved an orthopedic prosthesis, he referred the questions to me. It was like going through a residency program. With the exception of surgery, I was doing everything the residents were doing, and was receiving the same educational benefits. All this was thanks to Dr. Bruce Agee, who was not only a good doctor, but also a good person. He had genuine concern for his patients, a love of teaching, and scant interest in money or power. Nor is he the only doctor of his kind. I have discovered that most doctors, when approached by somebody who genuinely wants to learn, will go out of their way to be helpful.

On a quieter level, I was pursuing my medical education by reading medical journals and texts. I subscribed to the *Journal of Bone and Joint Surgery, Clinical Orthopaedics, Orthopedic Clinics of North America,* and *Surgery.* One of the first things I bought was a medical dictionary for fourteen dollars—I was amazed by the cost. After buying it, I realized it was useless until I learned enough medical terminology to understand it. About a week later, I was walking through a hospital lobby where a book salesman was selling medical volumes to doctors as they were leaving the hospital. I went over and bought both volumes of De Palma's *The Management of Fractures and Dislocations* plus some other orthopedic texts. I later bought the *Atlas of Orthopedic Surgery, The Textbook of Anatomy and Physiology,* and the *Manual of Internal Fixation.* The larger hospitals sometimes held book auctions to recycle old or extra volumes from their libraries. I once bought a copy of *Gray's Anatomy* for thirty-five cents at an auction. It was a 1950s edition, but I figured the human body has not changed since it was published.

I sat up nights and studied these sources, cramming as much as I could into my head. The biggest problem was making the words mean something. A book would describe the three points at which the surgeon drills holes into the acetabular cup during a total hip procedure: the ischium, the ilium, and the pubes—all foreign terms to me. So I wrote questions on three-by-five cards and carried them in my coat pocket. Whenever I found a friendly surgeon who really knew his business, I cornered him in the hallway or invited him for a cup of coffee. Then I asked him to illustrate the discussion on a napkin or scrap of paper. Thanks to dozens of helpful surgeons, my reading became more meaningful.

Unfortunately, the supply firm whose products I sold did far less to educate its salesmen. The company once held a two-day sales training seminar in the Midwest shortly after I joined it. The program included a color movie of the surgical implantation of a new total hip the company was introducing, plus a movie about a new total knee. I found the films educational because live surgery does not afford the same view inside the body as the camera. I later convinced my boss to buy some of these films and watched them, like a football coach, on weekends until I was thoroughly familiar with total knee and hip surgery.

Six months after I started selling the product line, the company sent me to the home office for a week-long seminar on soft goods. The program included discussions of slings, cervical collars, pelvic belts, abdominal binders, heel protectors, head frames, and traction equipment, but not of my favorite topics: joint implants and fracture appliances. A doctor lectured on skeletal anatomy, but at such a basic level that to me it seemed useless. Many salesmen attending the course, however, were new to the business and for them it was probably appropriate to call the femur the longest bone in the body, or the "leg bone." I found it dull.

Fortunately, the company also conducted a two-day course on internal bone fixation. A local butcher provided bones from freshly killed cows. We fractured the bones, which still had blood on them, then took surgical screwdrivers and drills, attached bone plates and screws, reunited the fractures, realigned bone fragments, and emerged better versed on the appliances we were trying to sell.

Meanwhile, my self-education program took an interesting turn. In late 1973 I witnessed a surgical procedure that proved to be memorable. George Schott, the real name of another medical supply salesman, had arranged for me to attend a craniotomy (brain surgery) at Smithtown General Hospital. I was very excited about it, but also apprehensive because I had never seen a craniotomy before. I remember asking George as we were driving to the hospital that morning, "Is this going to be bloody?" and he had said "No." I had deliberately skipped breakfast because I did not want to become nauseated (or worse) in the operating room.

George's role—which required that he be scrubbed—was to insure that a new drill the surgeons were using, a neurotome, worked properly. This nitrogen-driven turbine operates at speeds up to 20,000 rpm and, in this particular procedure, was fitted with a special drill bit to cut a half-inch hole in the skull. Using this trepanning hole as a starting point, the surgeons then could cut out a circular piece of skull cap with a blade resembling that of a Sabre saw. It represented a vast improvement over the previous technique in which the surgeon used a Gigli saw, or piece of wire with teeth on it and handles at each end. He would drill two or three trepanning holes in the skull, thread the wire through them and saw back and forth until the bone gave way. The Gigli left the skull cap in all sorts of irregular shapes instead of making the smooth, circular cut of the neurotome.

George and I arrived in the operating room before the two surgeons, Dr. Edward Altchek and Dr. Moses Ashkenazy, their real names. The patient was already anesthetized, and nurses were scurrying around carrying trays of sterile instruments, unwrapping the surgical sheets that covered them, and pouring sterile saline solution into the vats in which they wash instruments throughout the procedure. Suddenly Altchek and Ashkenazy made their entrance, the latter carrying a portable tape recorder under his arm. He placed it on a shelf in the corner of the room, and turned on acid-rock music.

I looked at George and whispered, "What's the music for?"

"These two guys like to have it when they're working," George said. "Breaks the monotony."

The surgeons left to scrub, returned about five minutes later, and started draping the patient's already shaven head with surgical sheets. (A surgeon usually does the draping because of the special techniques involved.) Dr. Ashkenazy told me to move closer for a better view. I was only a foot from the patient's head when he made the initial half-moon incision in the scalp. As the knife cut, I realized that I no longer related to the patient on the table as a person. The thought that kept going through my mind was that the patient's head looked just like a grapefruit. That image changed abruptly as the scalp was pulled back and the pale grapefruit suddenly turned bright red.

When the incision was completed and the skull laid bare, Dr. Ashkenazy picked up the neurotome and started to cut a circular piece of skull cap in order to expose the brain. He first drilled three trepanning holes in the skull, then exchanged the drill bit for an inch-and-a-half saw blade. At this point in the procedure, trouble struck. The blade jammed in the skull, causing Dr. Ashkenazy to look at the OR supervisor and ask, "What the hell's wrong? Why doesn't this thing work?" She turned to George, who was standing off to one side, and asked him to tell Ashkenazy how to handle the drill. George explained, and Dr. Ashkenazy resumed sawing. Again the blade jammed. The OR supervisor looked at George: "Why isn't it working?" He said, "Because he's holding it at the wrong angle." By then both surgeons were visibly upset. George explained that the blade must be held perpendicular to the skull so that it can move freely. After the saw blade lodged in the patient's head for the third time, Dr. Ashkenazy gave up and asked George to take over the drilling. George picked up the neurotome, freed the blade, held it at a right angle to the skull, and within a few minutes removed a piece of skull cap the diameter of an orange. He handed the neurotome back to Dr. Ashkenazy. It was the first time George had cut into a patient, although he had practiced many times on cadavers.

The next layer was the dura, a membrane that lies between the skull and brain. Ordinarily the surgeon cuts the dura with a scalpel after removing the skull cap. But in this case, Dr. Ashkenazy had torn about five inches of dura while holding the drill at the wrong angle. The bottom lip of the saw blade, which is supposed to peel the dura away from the skull, had caught the dura itself, ripping it along with the bone. Throughout the procedure, Dr. Altchek had been sealing off bleeding blood vessels with an electronic coagulating machine, the one that goes BZZZZZZZ. He stepped on the foot pedal, touched the end of each bleeder with a small probe, and burned it shut. At each pulse, the brain jumped.

George's participation in the case ended once the skull cap was removed. About ten minutes later, we walked out of the operating room while the case was still in progress, went to the doctor's lounge to change our clothes, thanked the OR supervisor for allowing me to observe, and left Smithtown General Hospital.

The entire experience gave me mixed emotions. First, I was aghast at the fact that George Schott, who is an orthopedic salesman and no more or no less, had laid hands on a patient during a craniotomy. My boss had said I would be involved in surgery, but I hardly thought *this* involved. What really astounded me was the lack of preparation for surgery. Here they were opening up a man's head and exposing the most vital and irreplaceable part of his body—the brain. And the surgeon, for starters, did not know how to operate the major piece of equipment used in this procedure.

As I learned later, many surgeons who are unfamiliar with this type of air drill make the same mistake as did Dr. Ashkenazy. It takes a number of cases for the surgeon to develop a feel for the instrument, and opportunities to practice are few. The problem was compounded at the time because there were no formal training programs available, and unless the doctors happened to try the air drill at a medical-meeting exhibit, their first experience with it was likely to occur when they used it on a patient.

The lack of professionalism I witnessed during that first craniotomy was appalling. I had seen so much good medical practice prior to this. Surely I had witnessed an aberration—or was it, perhaps, an omen of things to come? It was clear that if the latter proved true and I was going to spend time in surgery, I needed to be as well prepared as George to step in when needed. George had spent five years in the Navy as an operating-room and tissue-bank technician. There an OR technician does what an assistant surgeon does in the civilian world, so George's four hundred major and six hundred minor surgical procedures of all kinds represented an enormous wealth of experience. As a tissue-bank technician, George performed sterile postmortems, which resemble autopsies but are for the purpose of removing usable parts of the body—brains, arteries, skin, and other organs. The latter are freeze-dried and grafted to live patients many months later. The process is reminiscent of the best-selling book, *Coma,* except that instead of being victims of a vile murder plot, the patients are military personnel who have died natural deaths. I had none of George's vast experience, so I decided to accelerate my efforts at self-education.

Salesmen might go into surgery and hold a retractor or install a new attachment for a drill. But most did not know enough anatomy to tackle a skull cap as George had. They knew in theory, perhaps, but not in practice. A textbook could tell them that a prominence of bone is located at a certain point atop the femur. But when a surgeon feels for the prominence in a bleeding, open incision, it may be only in that general vicinity, not that exact spot. Surgery is a matter of feel, and the only way to learn it, I knew, was to reach inside an incision. I could not do that by watching operations or reading books. So I embarked upon the next, and final, phase of my medical self-education: I went to work on cadavers.

My first encounter with a dead body occurred soon after the craniotomy and two months after I began working in the emergency room. The chief orthopedic resident told me he and several colleagues planned to implant a total hip prosthesis in a cadaver.

"We're using your company's instruments," he said. "Do you want to come along?"

"I'd love to," I said.

As we walked downstairs to the morgue, it occurred to me that its very location, in a remote part of the hospital basement, symbolizes its lowly place in the medical community. The rest of the hospital staves off death. Only the morgue is at ease with its reality. Here death is accepted and even turned to positive purposes.

Although I was excited by the opportunity the chief resident had just offered, I was apprehensive about being confronted with a dead person. The sight that first greeted my eyes told me that the encounter would be stark and sudden. You cannot turn your eyes from the centerpiece of the morgue: an eight-foot steel table with a rim around the edge and a drain for blood and body fluids to flow through. I braced myself for a closer look. On the table, naked and unadorned except for a tan packaging tag tied to a left toe, was the body of a white male about sixty years old. On the tag were written his name and number, as if to acknowledge what a body is worth in death: allowing for inflation, some $2.70 worth of chemicals, it is said. But this lifeless form was infinitely more valuable now that it was about to teach us how to implant an artificial hip. The thought made it easier for me to approach the cadaver.

Two residents were waiting for us, perched on stools on either side of the table. We donned rubber gloves and plastic aprons like those that carpenters wear. I opened my case of Charnley total hip instruments, and one of the residents, discovering that some routine surgical tools were needed, called the operating room to send them down.

While waiting for the instruments, we hovered around the

body, crowding toward the hip area, leaning, gaping. No need to worry about breaking sterility here. The chief resident, to my surprise, asked me: "Do you want to make the initial incision?" I nodded eagerly, and he handed me the scalpel, laid his hand over mine, and showed me how to hold it. With my left hand I felt for the greater trochanter, landmark of total hip surgery, and started the incision about two inches above. At first I felt afraid, awed by the enormity of what I was about to do, and barely pressed with the scalpel.

"Go ahead, cut deeper, Bill. It's a long way to the hip capsule, so don't be afraid."

The cutting seemed endless, fascinating. My concentration was broken by the other residents: "Hey, this guy is dead!" "Hurry up." "We don't want to be here all night." For them, incisions were routine. They wanted to reach bone and try out the Charnley instruments.

Finally I reached the hip capsule. "All right, let's dislocate it," the chief resident said. We tried to pop the femoral head out of the socket by moving the cadaver's leg up toward the ceiling and rotating it, but the leg would not dislocate. So we sawed the femoral head and pried it from the socket with a shoehorn-type instrument called a bone skid, and started working on the hip. We drilled a pilot hole in the acetabulum to measure its thickness. We took turns reaming the hip socket with various instruments, experiencing their feel for the first time. We cemented in the acetabular cup, reamed out the femoral canal, and cemented in the lower half of the artificial hip. When, at last, the steel ball popped into the plastic hip socket, it felt like the final act of a dress rehearsal for a Broadway show.

This was my first cutting of human skin, although I had doctored horses during my equestrian days. I had used a scalpel at age fifteen when I gelded a horse, and later assisted at an operation to patch a hole in a horse's windpipe. But the experience in the autopsy room was another order of magnitude.

Several weeks after the cadaver hip implant, I attended an autopsy at another hospital. Two orthopedic residents planned to observe a postmortem and I asked if I could accompany them. "Sure," they said. In the morgue I stood at the foot of the dissecting table and watched a pathology resident ply his trade. He started his incision at the collarbone and, in one continuous stroke, cut all the way to the groin. He next peeled back the flesh and laid the entire chest and abdomen open with hooks the size of a curved index finger. They were embedded in the skin down the sidelines of the body. Then, to my utter horror, he picked up a hammer—not a surgical mallet but a common carpenter's hammer—and broke the ribs away.

I was so shocked by this unspeakable invasion of another person's body that I resolved, on the spot, that none of my loved ones—no matter what the circumstances of their deaths—would ever be subjected to an autopsy if I could help it.

The pathology resident next removed the left lung, the only organ, as I recall, that he wanted. The other two residents were learning how to approach the spine from the front during spinal surgery, a procedure that requires major rearrangement of the abdominal organs. They also cut away small slivers of various organs to make slides for tissue studies. When everybody had extracted his ounce, or pound, of flesh, the pathologist gathered up the ribs he had broken and tossed them, helter-skelter, back into the body cavity. He removed the skin hooks, took a needle and suture, made about thirteen fast stitches, and literally slammed the chest back together, one, two, three. I felt totally repulsed.

Meanwhile I had, since starting selling, been buying cadaver bones from several special mail-order houses. I could buy a small femur for about seven dollars, a medium one for eight, and a large one for about ten. Actually, all the bones were smaller than the average American's, because they came from India and other Asian countries where bodies are easy to obtain.

An assembled skeleton cost about five hundred dollars, but I bought a disarticulated one for two hundred less. When it arrived, I took the box of bones to my garage and laid them out on the floor, identified them, and rearranged them in their proper positions. I found the metatarsals, the cuneiforms, and the navicular bones and put the right foot together. I gathered the vertebrae and put the spine together. In the body these bones are held together by muscles, tendons, and tissue, but I had to use wire. Suddenly skeletal anatomy became very logical: I could see the way God designed the pieces to interlock and interface with one another. Some people might compare it to putting an Erector set together, but an Erector set fits in many different ways. There is only one way to assemble a skeleton.

The bones did not entirely meet my needs, however. When I

35

tried to saw or nail them and implant a hip or knee prosthesis, they were so dry that they shattered in my hands. Then one day I was talking to some residents at a hospital who had just amputated a woman's leg. The leg was in a plastic bag on a stretcher outside the operating room, awaiting a porter who would carry it down to the incinerator room. Suddenly it dawned on me that this leg had a femur, a tibia, a fibula, a patella, a complete foot. What impressed me most, as I felt the bag, was that the hip end of the femur was totally intact. A dynamite leg! I had to have it. I asked one of the residents if I could take it, and he said, "No way! You can never get your hands on that. We incinerate amputated legs because they're probably dirty." By dirty, he meant infected.

I told myself, "Keep quiet, Bill, and follow that leg downstairs." I chatted with the resident until the porter arrived, then excused myself and followed the leg to the subbasement of the hospital. The porter pushed it as far as the incinerator-room door and, to my utter joy, left it there on the stretcher. I raced out to the parking lot and opened my car trunk, where I kept a heavy-duty plastic trash bag for slings, braces, and the like. I dumped everything out and walked back carrying it in my pocket.

When I reached the subbasement, the leg was still there. I tried to bend it at the knee, but it was becoming stiff. I struggled for a while, finally fit my bag over it diagonally, and left the hospital via the boiler room and a rear loading platform. As I stuffed the bag into the trunk of my car, I thought, "Oh boy, I'm going to take this leg apart!" I could not continue working that day because in a few hours the leg would have started smelling bad. So I drove home to Stony Brook, and asked my wife for the roasting pan she uses to cook turkey. She said, "What do you want it for?" "Never mind," I replied, and stepped into the two-car garage that was attached to the house.

A few minutes later, a neighbor came over and asked what I was doing. My booty was still in the bag, and I told him I was going to dissect a leg. He did not believe me until I opened the bag. He stood in the far corner of the garage and watched as I grabbed the flesh with a rake retractor, cut it away with a disposable scalpel, and threw the cuttings into the bag. By the time I finished, the neighbor had disappeared. I put the bones, except for the foot and talus, which I did not need, into the roasting pan, which was not really big enough for the job. I then went to the kitchen for a gallon jug of Clorox, poured it into the roasting pan, and covered the top with plastic wrap to let it soak overnight. The next morning I scrubbed the bones with a wire brush to remove the remaining flesh.

Then I asked another friend, who is in the chemical business, for something to bleach the bones. He gave me an unmarked glass bottle containing some nameless concoction, which I poured in with the Clorox. The brew gurgled and smoked, and when I returned to the garage two hours later, the bones were bleached a beautiful yellow-white. I hung them from wire coathangers to let them dry for a few days, then put various implants in them.

Thus began a strange alliance. The tradeoff was this: my friend provided the chemicals I needed, in infinite variety, and I gave him the opportunity to become the handmaiden, as it were, of science. He would arrive at my back door, bottle in hand. "What do you have this time?" I would ask when we were safe in the privacy of my garage.

He never told me what was in his chemical creations. But he would ask: "Do you think I could sell this stuff to the medical schools?" Or: "How's that stuff I brought over yesterday? Did it do a better job of cleaning the bones?" At times he was positively ghoulish, but I could not help responding to his enthusiasm.

As time passed, his concoctions became, if not better, certainly more spectacular. Once he brought me a solution that burned the bristles off a toothbrush I was using to scour a bone. Another time, I made the mistake of adding household ammonia to the latest batch he had brought over. I was trying to remove the flesh from a foot I was holding with a long set of clamps. Suddenly, the contents of the turkey pan started to smolder. Fumes curled upward. My eyes watered. I decided to remove the foot, lest I completely dissolve it. Then a worse thought occurred: "My God, I'm going to blow up the garage!" I considered neutralizing the brew with baking soda, but stopped myself and realized that, with my knowledge of chemistry, I could have blown up my house.

At the end of a bone-cleaning session, I would empty the flesh I had removed into a double layer of plastic trash bags, spray inside with a disinfectant, and tie them in tight knots so that the sanitation men would not become curious about the contents. I could just imagine them finding a foot, half stripped of its flesh, and telling the police that an axe murderer was disposing of bodies from his home in Stony Brook. Once the bones were bleached and dried, I was home free.

In time, I acquired another accomplice in my bone-collecting endeavors, a salesman I will call Wolf, who worked for another medical-equipment company. A competitor by day, Wolf was my able assistant by night. We used to practice for hours drilling holes in bones, implanting artificial joints, attaching screws, nails, and all manner of orthopedic paraphernalia. One day our activities, strictly amateur until now, suddenly turned commercial. A vice president from his company had seen an Austin-Moore hip prosthesis his company made implanted into a femur. The executive asked who did the implant, and Wolf, a shrewd soul, quickly sensed that his answer might prove profitable.

"Oh, I have a friend who does them for me."

"If we give you one hundred femurs, can you get your friend to do them for us? I'd like to give one to all our salesmen."

"I'll talk to him," said Wolf, shrewd to the end. That night he came over.

"Bill, I've got a great deal. We're going to make five hundred dollars!"

"Doing what?" I said.

"The company's giving me a hundred femurs, and all we have to do is cut off the necks, rasp them out, and insert Austin-Moores. They'll pay us five dollars a femur!"

That may not have proved profitable on a one-for-one basis, but we decided to mass-produce them. About a week later we received a huge box of femurs. We took them to Wolf's garage, where—thanks to his radial saw—I removed about a dozen femoral heads per minute. Soon the floor was littered with them. Meanwhile, Wolf took the femurs and rasped them to the size and shape of an Austin-Moore prosthesis. We finished the job in one evening, and made $250 apiece. Now we had one hundred femoral heads.

"What will we do with these?" Wolf asked.

"Let's save them. They must have some use."

About eight months later I was talking to a doctor in Queens who said, "I'd love to find a bunch of femoral heads for some cross-section studies."

"How many do you need?" I asked.

"As many as I can get."

"How much would you offer for a hundred of them?"

"Two hundred dollars," he said.

"You write the check, I'll deliver the heads," I told him.

So we sold the femoral heads and ended up making $700 on the entire project.

One of our more interesting enterprises was acquiring a cadaver. An arm or leg was relatively simple to obtain, but when I helped implant the total hip in the morgue, I learned how hard cadavers are to come by. One day I heard that a medical school had just donated not one, but two, cadavers to a hospital in the Bronx. An event like this so excites the typical resident that he talks about it like a youngster with a new bike. I decided to check the cadavers out. There was a male and a female. The next day I was at the hospital where I worked with Dr. Agee's residents. I owed these gentlemen a favor for having taught me so much, and for months they had wanted a cadaver. So I said, "I know where I can get you one."

"Come on, how are you going to get a cadaver?" replied Frank, as I will call the chief resident.

"I found one at a hospital in another county. Do you want a male or female? I can grab either one."

"Grab?" Frank said.

"Yes, I'm going to *swipe* a cadaver! You want to take a ride with me tonight?"

Frank did, and I arranged to pick him up around six o'clock for a spaghetti dinner at an Italian restaurant. I ordered a lot of wine because I wanted to prepare him for the stresses of what we would be doing. I had made other preparations as well: in the back of my nine-passenger Chevy Caprice station wagon was a pair of white coveralls from a food-processing plant.

After dinner we drove to the hospital and went directly to the morgue, which fortunately was not locked. Lining the walls were dozens of doors about two feet square, with handles like those on refrigerators in a chain-store meat department. I knew from my previous visit which two doors I wanted. The male body was behind the first door and, as usual, it slid out on a roller. I asked Frank whether he wanted the man or the woman.

"What does she look like?" he asked. I opened the door and pulled her out.

"Let's take the man."

I pushed her back in, and we carried the male cadaver to the steel dissecting table against one wall of the room. It was not difficult to put the coveralls on him. His body was so full of embalming fluid that it was not stiff. When our friend was dressed, I told Frank to wait. I left and returned with a wheelchair, steering past several scrub buckets on wheels scattered around the floor. We sat the cadaver in the chair and wheeled him down the hall to the back loading platform.

"Stay here," I told Frank. "Nobody will question you."

I backed my station wagon up to the platform. Frank wanted to lay the cadaver in the back, but I said that would raise suspicion. So we propped him in the front seat and attached the shoulder harness and seat belt. He sat there with his head tilted back, looking at the ceiling of the car. As an added touch, I draped his left arm across the back of the seat.

The next obstacle was the toll gate on the bridge. I was headed for the exact-change lane when I discovered I did not have seventy-five cents in coins. By now I was also feeling confident, so I pulled up to the toll booth and handed the attendant a five-dollar bill. As he leaned to hand me change, he glanced inside the car. I grinned and, by the expression on his face, *I knew he knew* he was looking at a dead man. Frank and I then drove to the hospital to deliver the cadaver to Dr. Agee's residents, who were so grateful they talked about it for months. Sometime later I was talking to the residents at the hospital where the cadaver came from.

"Gee," one of them said, "did you hear that somebody swiped our cadaver? Stealing dead bodies—what's it coming to?"

"That's terrible," I said. "But you still have the other one, right?"

"Yeah, we still have the other one."

And, until this writing, they never learned who stole their cadaver.

Sometimes I would only borrow a body. For example, in September 1977 a doctor on the staff of a private hospital mentioned that they had had a number of deaths lately. "How many are in the freezer right now?" I asked him. He told me.

"You got any that nobody cares about?"

"We've got a woman," he said. "We're having trouble getting the family to pick up the body."

"Do you think they'd mind if I try something out with a total knee? After I finish I'll close up, and nobody will ever know unless they start checking the knees."

"All right," he said, "only I don't want to know anything about it. And don't mutilate the body."

So about ten o'clock one night an associate and I implanted a total knee my company sold. When we finished, I put about fourteen stitches in the knee. From the coroner's report, the undertaker would know the knee was opened after the woman died, but he would probably assume that, for one reason or another, a doctor had opened the knee to check something out.

My cadaver work continued as long as I sold medical equipment, for dead bodies were always in great demand among my customers. Whenever I needed a cadaver for a hospital where I did business, I would pay a midnight visit to a certain medical examiner's office. There, for a case of Red Label, an amiable morgue attendant would slip a John Doe into the back of my station wagon and cover it with a tarp. I would drive it to some appreciative residents in a hospital in the greater New York City area where my business, in the forthcoming year, could be expected to increase by at least fifty percent.

On the other hand, every time I scrubbed with a doctor during surgery, my business in that institution would increase even more. And since surgical cases were more plentiful than cadavers, I began to steer my medical career in new directions.

FOUR

HANDS ON

The first time I ever touched a patient was in 1974 during the surgical installation of an artificial knee—a total knee arthroplasty. Given the unorthodox nature of my medical education, I was as ready as could be expected for it. One February afternoon, I visited an orthopedic surgeon in my territory to tell him about the different implants I sold and to persuade him to switch to my product line. On that particular day, he had something to sell me. He had a daughter who worked for him, an attractive girl in her early twenties, and as I sat talking to him—I did not wear a wedding band in those days—I could see the idea take shape. He called for a patient's file, and when she brought it into the room, he made his move: "Oh, honey, do you know Bill MacKay?" As soon as she left, he said, "You married, Bill?"

"Yeah, I've got a couple of kids."

"Oh."

I could see the matchmaker's anticipation drain from his face. Now he was ready really to talk business. It was a ritual that was becoming all too familiar, and it began something like this:

"I have a candidate for a total hip. I'm scheduling this patient for three weeks from today. Bring me all the literature because I haven't decided which hip to use yet."

He tells this to four different salesmen, and the one who seems smartest and most knowledgeable sells the hip. When I bring him the prosthesis, however, I cannot say, "I know you've never done a total hip but don't worry, I'll get you through the case." I never ask, "Are you going to use my prosthesis?" I am tactful and positive:

"Doctor, let me make a suggestion. I'll go over to the hospital and in-service the nurses so they'll be familiar with the instruments and know *how we are going to do this case.*"

Then I give him the big laminga, as I call it.

"We both know that when I give an in-service, only about ten percent of the nurses pay attention. And about ten percent of that ten percent comprehend what I'm talking about. So let me make this suggestion: suppose I come in on the case and make sure the nurses hand you the proper instruments, since it's the first total hip we've done at this hospital."

"Oh, have you been in on these before?"

"Doctor, I go in on total hips all the time!"

"Oh." Suddenly he looks at me like I am the Great White Hope. To himself he says, "He can talk me through this case." Thus the basic deal is struck.

Having accepted the veiled invitation in this case, to help implant an artificial knee, I spent the next few days reading up on the procedure. It is an exacting one that requires considerable drilling, sawing, and chiseling of bone to fit the contours of the prosthesis. The procedure also required something I did not think of until several days later: "I'm going to the scrub sink with this surgeon, but I've never actually scrubbed because I've never touched a patient." When that day came, I knew, my hands had better be clean. I decided to learn how to scrub, and called a friendly nurse who was operating-room supervisor at a hospital in my territory.

"I've got a problem," I told her. "I have to scrub in with a doctor, and the truth of the matter is I really don't know how to scrub. Would you teach me?"

Gladys, I will call her, said, "Sure, I'm quitting work at three o'clock. Pick me up then, and I'll teach you how to scrub."

At 3 P.M. I arrived at the operating-room area just as she was walking out.

"Can you give me a ride to my apartment?" she asked.

As I drove her home, I wondered whether she planned to teach me to scrub there. When we arrived she asked me to sit down, relax, and have a drink while she changed clothes. The way things were happening, the way she was moving around the apartment, I knew she was looking to do more than teach me how to scrub. Meanwhile, I was being very straight about the whole thing. I could see she was getting frustrated by the situation, but she was not willing to admit what she wanted. Finally, she said, "Come on, let's go back to the hospital. Everybody is probably gone now, and I can teach you how to scrub."

When we returned to the hospital, the main door to the operating-room area was locked. She found the key, unlocked it, and we went in. "Go into the doctor's lounge and put on scrub clothes," she said. This seemed unnecessary, and I said so. "I want to teach you how to scrub right. Go put on scrub clothes, please." She was really dragging it out. "All right," I said to myself, but I was looking at my watch because I had a six o'clock appointment with a doctor in Bayside, and it was already after four. I changed into scrub clothes and when I came out I discovered that she had changed too: into a scrub nurse's dress with snaps all the way down the front. Only she had not bothered to snap it. At that point I knew there were only two things I could do, and I did not want to run. So we made it on a stretcher, right there in the operating room!

It was after five o'clock when she finally introduced me to the surgical ritual of scrubbing. She showed me how to open the little aluminum package that holds the sterile sponge with its backing of plastic bristles. She taught me how to build up the orange lather of antiseptic Betadine surgical soap in the sponge side, and work the brush in a direction away from my wrist, scrubbing under the nails, across the knuckles, around the fingertips, between the fingers, up the arm, all the way to the elbow. Then open another brush and scrub every square inch of the other hand and arm. It was a ten-minute handwash that would make any American mother proud.

But Gladys was not yet satisfied. "Now," she said, "take the brush and throw it in the trash. Hold your hands toward the ceiling, step on the foot pedal, and rinse so that the water runs away from your hands and off the elbow." I followed directions. She was pleased with my performance.

44

"Your hands," she smiled, "are sterile. Don't touch any-thing. The scrub nurse will hand you a sterile towel and help you into surgical gloves, and you'll be ready to operate." Gladys had taught me the double-brush technique, using one scrub brush for each hand. Some surgeons use the single-brush technique, but the other is better. What Gladys showed me that day served me well in later years. For one thing, I never had an operating-room supervisor or doctor complain about the way I scrubbed.

On the morning of the total knee case, I went to the operating room of the same hospital and met the surgeon—I will call him Dr. Carl Gilford—and in the doctor's lounge he intro-duced me to Dr. Jim Mikeska, who was going to assist at the operation. Mikeska, as I call him, was a big, heavyset man with coarse manners and a way of hurrying through life. He was not particularly cordial to me because he had wanted to use another company's total knee in the procedure. Dr. Gilford showed me to a locker: "Put your clothes in there and your money in your sock." Doctor's lounges, he reminded me, are prime targets for thieves. I pinned my wrist watch to my shirt, put on a two-piece green scrub suit, and went to the sinks. When the operating-room supervisor asked me "Do you know how to scrub?" I thought to myself, "If you only knew!" I scrubbed like a veteran, entered the operating room, and put on gown and gloves.

The patient, an elderly woman with severe arthritis of the knee, was already anesthetized, and after some discussion with Dr. Mikeska about where to make the knee incision, Dr. Gilford took a scalpel and prepared to cut. The knee was covered with Vidrape and propped at a 90-degree angle over some rolled-up surgical sheets. Midway up the thigh bone, a tourniquet hose encircled the leg and connected to a small box hanging from a metal intravenous stand.

When Dr. Gilford was ready to make his incision, a ten-inch gash down the middle of the knee, he told the circulating nurse to turn on the tourniquet. She flipped a switch which caused a bottle of aerosol to fill the tourniquet hose and restrict the blood flow. As the resulting pounds of pressure constricted the leg, a time clock, in essence, was set on the procedure. After about an hour, the surgeon would release the tourniquet, or else the lower leg would start to die from lack of oxygen-carrying blood. He would disconnect the tourniquet about two minutes, reapply it, dry out the wound, and resume the operation.

Some surgeons can implant an artificial knee so fast that

they never need to release the tourniquet. Dr. Gilford, however, was a careful man who believed in taking time to do a good job. With great deliberation, he laid the knee joint bare, exposing the lower end of the femur and upper end of the tibia or shin bone. He moved the kneecap (patella) off to the side and secured it with a clamp. Throughout this process, Dr. Gilford stood at the patient's right, Dr. Mikeska was across the table, and the scrub nurse was at the foot. I stood to her left, near the instrument table, and watched.

Surgical replacement of the knee joint was an exciting enterprise in the early 1970s, when this operation took place. Although the first successful artificial knees were already twenty years old, a new type of knee, incorporating many of the advances Dr. John Charnley had already made in hip technology, was not introduced until 1971. Most of the knee work took place at Mayo and Cleveland clinics and the Hospital for Special Surgery in New York City. At this early stage, total knee arthroplasty was best left to highly skilled surgeons in preeminent institutions that could handle large numbers of cases.

Far more complicated than the hip, the knee is a hinged joint that rolls, glides, and rotates in only one plane, but with infinite centers of rotation. The twin skids of the femoral component slide back and forth in the mated grooves of the tibial component to simulate the knee's natural action, whereas the ball part of the artificial hip rolls in all planes inside the acetabular cup.

Why, then, were some minor-league surgeons attempting this procedure, which is far more difficult than implanting a total hip? For one reason, whenever medical advances take place, patients hear about them and pressure their doctors—in communities large and small—to give them the latest artificial hip, knee, or elbow. Many doctors succumb to the pleadings of humans in pain, and to the dictates of their own egos, which lure them into big-league surgery. Plus (and here I share the responsibility) there are the blandishments of the marketplace. At least three dozen types of artificial knees had already been designed at the time (more than eighty are available today in the United States and abroad) and I, as a medical-equipment salesman, was interested in promoting the cause of total knees in general, and my company's brand in particular.

Thus Dr. Gilford, to whom I had sold a total knee, stood in the operating room one spring day in 1974. He began transforming the lower end of the femur from its natural rounded shape to sharply angled planes that would exactly fit the stems, grooves, and dovetails of the upper half of the knee prosthesis. Dr. Gilford first sawed off the condyles, twin knobs on the lower end of the femur. To aid in the cutting, he used a template that fitted over the uncut bone and told him where to direct his tools.

More sculptor than surgeon, Dr. Gilford worked cautiously, knowing that if the cuts were too deep, too shallow, incorrectly angled, or if the knee were otherwise improperly installed, the patient might be unable to straighten her leg after surgery. Or the leg might refuse to bend, or wobble from side to side so that she could not stand on it. Or the patella might click against the prosthesis and cause pain. The leg might have to be fused— surgically welded into a straight position. It might end up two inches shorter than the other leg, requiring the patient to wear a thick heel. Or, worst of all, the leg might have to be amputated.

Mindful of these consequences, Dr. Gilford completed his handiwork, removing one small piece of bone at a time, chiseling with the osteotome, snipping here and there with rongeurs, surgical pliers with sharp cutting ends. With painstaking care, he fashioned the femur into a mirror image of the cutting jig. When, at last, he looked up from his task, I knew I was in the presence of a true craftsman whose work few eyes were privileged to see, for soon it would be hidden under the femoral prosthesis.

I was enthralled by the process, but Dr. Mikeska's body language indicated that he wanted to hurry things along. For example, he periodically looked at me, then up at the ceiling in mock exasperation. But Dr. Gilford was not to be hurried. Bone still needed to be removed from between the femoral condyles to accommodate the bridge of the prosthesis. He approached the area with a small osteotome and mallet. When he was finished, the dummy prosthesis did not quite fit. He removed it and trimmed more bone.

Now it came time to prepare the tibia for the lower half of the artificial knee. Dr. Gilford began carving it in the same manner as he had the femur. Suddenly Dr. Mikeska, who had been holding retractors, suctioning blood, and performing the usual duties of an assistant surgeon, lost what remained of his patience: "Come on. Can't you take more bone off?"

Dr. Gilford ignored him and continued at his own pace. Suddenly, Dr. Mikeska seized an osteotome and said, "Let me do this damn thing. Come on, we're wasting too much time." And before the other surgeon could stop him or even protest, Dr. Mikeska smashed the instrument into the top of the tibia, shattering and breaking away the inside portion.

"What did you do that for?" Dr. Gilford demanded.

"For Christ sake," Dr. Mikeska answered, "we'll fill it in with cement. I can't spend all day on this. I figured we'd be here two hours."

"You damn near ruined her knee!" Dr. Gilford replied, without ever raising his voice. But his eye language and tone were deafening. Never before had I seen two surgeons at odds. Had they both carried guns, it would have been a rerun of the shootout at the OK Corral. They were furious with one another, and each thought he was equally right. Without another word, Dr. Mikeska turned and stomped out of the room.

Dr. Gilford turned to me: "Give me a hand, will you?"

"Sure, Doctor."

"What do you think I ought to do," he asked. "I have the whole medial side broken away here, and we don't have any asymmetric tibial plateaus." (This type of prosthesis is thicker on one side than the other, and would have been ideally suited for the situation.)

"Doctor," I said, "I think you should take the bone fragment that Dr. Mikeska broke out, put a bone screw through it, and reattach it to the tibia."

"Okay," he said. "If it doesn't work, we can always build up the area with cement."

Thus the moment arrived when I first touched a patient during surgery. The act was ordinary enough. I held retractors, something any intern would do, while Dr. Gilford tried on the tibial prosthesis to see how much bone was missing. At his request, I took a mallet and removed the prosthesis, tapping lightly and using hardly any force at all. For the next hour and twenty minutes, the two of us carefully trimmed rough edges off the broken bone fragment, shaping it to fit back on the tibia. I drilled it with a small hand drill, and Dr. Gilford held the fragment in place while I inserted a cancellous screw designed to hold soft and spongy interior bone. Dr. Gilford took a bone file and slowly rasped the top of the tibial plateau to make it even with the other side. He then inserted the femoral component, and we moved the patient's lower leg to check for stability and alignment of the knee.

It moved from full extension to a 90-degree angle; the

normal knee is capable of 135 degrees of flexion. The patient would never do yoga again, if indeed she ever had, and the surgery might cramp her lovemaking style. On the other hand, she would be able to negotiate stairs and this—aside from the absence of pain—is the ultimate test of the success or failure of a total knee. Before surgery she could hardly bend the leg at all.

After removing both components of the prosthesis, Dr. Gilford released the tourniquet for two minutes, rinsed the wound with an antibiotic, dried it with gauze, and repositioned the prosthesis for a final check. The scrub nurse mixed methyl-methacrylate cement and handed it to Dr. Gilford, who pushed it into the shaft of the femur and the underside of the prosthesis. He held it in place until the cement hardened. He then tempo-rarily inserted the tibial component to be sure it still fit, now that cement had been added to the femur. Dr. Gilford worked cement into the tibial bed and undersurface of the prosthesis, inserting it for the final time. The leg was fully extended while the cement set. I held the tibial component between my thumb and ring finger to keep it from twisting, knowing that if the knee prosthesis ever failed, it would probably be because the tibial component had worked loose.

When it came time to sew the patient's knee back together, a new problem became apparent. Dr. Mikeska, in the act of smashing the upper corner of the tibia, had cut through the patellar ligament that runs down the center front of the knee. This tendon holds the kneecap in place and stabilizes the knee joint. Dr. Gilford stretched the ligament and stapled it about two inches down the tibia, taking up some slack. He finished sewing up the patient and left two Hemovac tubes in place to drain blood from the wound during the next twenty-four hours. As we left the operating room, Dr. Gilford said, "I really appreciate your being here today, Bill. You were a tremendous help. If I can do anything for you in the future, let me know." I said, "Doctor, I'm just glad I could be of assistance."

I left the hospital that day with a feeling that bordered on euphoria. I had sawed bones on the carpenter's table of my garage. I had implanted artificial joints in cadavers—and stolen the bodies to do it. I had handled emergencies with residents. I had witnessed surgery. I had attended a case where another salesman cut off the tip of a patient's skull. But this was different. This was the first time I assisted in a case. Even though my role was relatively small, I helped solve the problem of how to repair the broken tibia. I helped make the idea work with my own hands. The entire experience was the turning point in my career as a medical-equipment salesman. From the moment I laid hands on a patient for the first time, I knew that surgery—not just watching, not just holding retractors, not just handling or assembling instruments, but *hands-on* surgery was what I wanted to do.

FIVE

DOING IT

As far back as I can remember, I always wanted to be a doctor. I had long admired and respected doctors, and the roots of this admiration sprang from a physician I had known since childhood. His name was Dr. Francis H. Keckeissen and he grew up in Queens, where he and my father were boyhood friends. They parted ways when Frank went to medical school and became chief surgeon at St. Vincent's Hospital in New York City, but their friendship was renewed later on, and he became our family doctor. As a child, I always thought he looked and acted as a doctor should. He was tall, athletically built, extroverted, sophisticated. He dressed impeccably in the style of the time: three-button tweed suits, rep ties, wing-tipped shoes. The inner man appealed to me even more. He always had time for me, and took genuine interest in what I was doing. With a waiting room full of patients, he would sit and talk doctor talk to me, show me his medical books, and answer my child's questions as we turned the pages.

Dr. Keckeissen had a wonderful bedside manner as well. I once developed a case of abdominal cramps that my parents were

51

convinced was appendicitis. My father drove me to Dr. Keckeissen's office in the Bronx. He examined me thoroughly: "No, it's not appendicitis. What you've got, Billy, is green-apple cramps." He died several years ago, but I admired that man more than any other person in the world.

I used to tell Dr. Keckeissen about wanting to become a doctor, and he always encouraged me. Becoming a doctor meant going to medical school, however, and schooling had never been one of my happier experiences. During seventh grade, for example, I wrote a sixteen-page paper on the heart and its functions. The teacher failed me because she said it was impossible for a seventh-grader to have written such a paper. Dr. Keckeissen had loaned me his copy of *Gray's Anatomy* as my source of information about the heart. And I had done a drawing showing the four chambers of the heart, and the bicuspid, tricuspid, and the aortic valves that regulate the blood flow from one chamber to the next. I protested the teacher's decision by quitting Garden City Junior High School. It was springtime, and I had completed enough of the year so that they graduated me from seventh grade. The following year I attended three different schools in eighth grade. The final break with formal education came after the fourth day of ninth grade, when I caused an uproar during algebra class and was suspended. These experiences ended my hopes of ever attending medical school.

But my medical *career* was far from over. Following the total knee case with Dr. Gilford and Dr. Mikeska, when I first touched a patient, I became more deeply involved in orthopedics—from simple traction to the most complex total hip surgery. At a simpler level, I applied splints, braces, casts, and ordinary traction. Brace-fitting I learned by experience. A general practitioner who wanted to put knee braces on an eleven-year-old boy sent me to the child's home in Queens. I remember feeling very nervous about this because I was not a professional brace-fitter, was new in the business, and might fit the devices wrong. There I stood in this child's living room, while his mother and father sat on the couch, thinking I was a pro. I tape-measured the child's calf, knee, and lower thigh, went to my car and pulled the right-size brace, according to the measurements, from my trunk. It was just like fitting shoes, only higher up.

I learned traction by reading a few books and watching technicians do it in the hospital. Although traction is surrounded by mystique, it is a very inexact science. The consequences can be serious if a patient is put in traction improperly. But the doctor usually changes the weights and pulleys in time, because the patient hurts badly enough.

One of my early experiences with traction occurred one day when I called on the emergency room of a hospital. Ambulances were bringing in casualties after a serious automobile accident. Suddenly the emergency room was filled with youngsters in pain. Because the facility was shorthanded at the time, the attending surgeon asked me to help out. We took one child, whose thigh bone had broken in midshaft, to the operating room, gave her a local anesthetic, and hand-drilled a hole through her femur just above the knee. We inserted a Steinmann pin through the drill hole. It is a narrow steel rod, about nine inches long and three-sixteenths of an inch in diameter, that protrudes on both sides of the leg so that weights can be attached. This process, known as skeletal traction, stretches the muscles, which contract when a person breaks a leg, aligns the bones, and prevents them from overriding one another. By releasing the tension on the muscles, ligaments, and tendons, skeletal traction allows nature to set the bone. Afterward, I remember taking this little girl to her room and meeting her mother and father. To this day they think I was a doctor.

Sometimes I encountered doctors who knew absolutely nothing about setting up traction and who would ask, "Hey, Mac, will you show me how to set this frame?"

In 1973, a doctor had me put a woman with a fractured pelvis into a Weil pelvic sling. He planned to leave her in traction several days and then put her in a cast. When I entered her room, she spewed forth the foulest, most vulgar language I have ever heard in my life. I finally told her, "Look, I don't work here, and I don't have to put up with your bullshit. Lie still and shut up or you're going to hurt all night because I'll walk out of here and leave you." She quieted down, and I put her in the sling. Four days later she was taken to the operating room for a cast. I never learned why, but somebody decided to shave her pubic area. When this happened, she started screaming and cursing so loudly that she could be heard three blocks away. The doctor was visibly upset. Finally I quieted her down, and we put the body cast on her, trimming it around her hips. I ended up visiting her several times a week while she was hospitalized, because I was one of the few people who could communicate with her, and keep her from going totally berserk.

One of the fascinations of the orthopedic business was the patients. For example, a hospital once called me to order an extra-large rib belt for a woman with a large barrel. The belt is elastic with cutouts for the woman's breasts, and it applies pressure around the rib cage so that during breathing, it acts as a splinting mechanism and reduces the pain. I went to the directress of nursing's office with the belt, and she said, "Oh, yes, you're the supply man. Come on, we'll go see the patient." We rode the elevator to a room occupied by two women. One was very good-looking; the other weighed at least 250 pounds and looked like Elsie the Cow. Needless to say, I wanted to put the belt on the good-looking woman, but it was for Elsie. I struggled with the belt, trying to slide it under her back, while she groaned. "Oh, don't move me, don't move me." I assume she suffered from low back pain, which is common with obese people. Finally I positioned the belt under her and told the nurse (who must be present whenever a male works with a female patient) to lift her gown so I could connect the rib belt. As the nurse complied, I stood there, stunned. Never in my life had I even imagined a pair of breasts that large. It was awesome. I looked at the directress of nursing, who gave me a "yeah-I-know" look. I fastened the rib belt, which was six inches wide and was like trying to cover a total hip incision with a Band-aid. But that is what the doctor wanted.

Doctors wanted me for more than setting up traction. The requests came couched in orders for artificial joints, bone plates, compression screws and, of course, the instruments for installing them. The hospital usually borrowed the instruments, especially for new procedures that were experimental and not likely to become part of that hospital's surgical repertory. If an orthopedist liked a particular hip and began using it frequently, the hospital might invest $4500 for the instruments. But some hospitals I dealt with, even after four years, never bought their own instruments even though the staff performed as many as twenty-five total hip procedures. Despite the fact that it borrowed Charnley hip instruments at least a dozen times during the two years I sold supplies there, one hospital never purchased a set. And as long as the hospital did not own the instruments, the surgeons could not perform a particular procedure unless I or another salesman brought them in. Several days would pass before I could retrieve the instruments, because the nurses had to clean and repack them in a surgical tray.

Invitations for my presence during surgery were also

couched in requests for an "in-service" to familiarize the operating-room nurses with instruments to be used during the case. The preceding day, or perhaps early in the morning before surgery, I would spend half an hour in the nurses' lounge explaining what each instrument was, its purpose, and when it would be used during the case. I would then be expected to stay for the case to make sure the nurses remembered what I had just told them. And once in the operating room I would be expected to pass instruments, hold retractors—and more, if the need arose.

A typical case illustrates how I was drawn, by a doctor's wishes, circumstances, and my own willingness, into the role of ghost surgeon. One day the secretary for two surgeons I will call Charles Singletary and Norman Lesher called my house and left word that the latter had a total hip procedure booked. The doctor wanted to know would I deliver the prosthesis and instruments to the hospital, and would I be free on the day of surgery? On the morning of the case, I arrived at the hospital where they practiced at around seven-fifteen and went to the doctor's lounge. I dressed in greens, foot covers, a cap and double masks, leaving the latter hanging around my neck. I never bothered to ask who the patient was.

As I walked down the hall toward the operating room, I saw the patient lying on a stretcher in the corridor. "Holy Christ," I thought. "I know this guy!" I quickly pulled up my mask because I had no idea how he would react to my presence. I hovered at the end of the hall, wishing the anesthesiologist would hurry up and put him to sleep. Finally I said to myself, "All right, what the hell, I can't stall any longer." I adjusted my mask and started down the hall. About ten feet past his stretcher, which was to the right of the corridor, I heard, in a deep Irish broque, "Bill . . ." I thought, "Oh, shit, he's spotted me. Now I have to turn around and talk to him." So I removed my mask and said, "Hi, Mike, how are you?"

"What are you doing here, Bill?"

"I'm just working with the doctors. I sell for one of the companies that makes the products they're using."

"Oh, are you going to be there during my surgery?"

"Well, I'm going to be around."

"Oh, great, Bill. How tough is this procedure? Is everything going to be okay?"

"Sure, Mike, don't worry about it. You'll be fine."

At that moment a nurse came and pushed him into the operating room where the anesthesiologist put him to sleep. The case started like most Charnley procedures, but it was unusual in one respect because the patient was in his thirties. The life expectancy of a total hip prosthesis is ten to fifteen years, so they are seldom implanted in a patient under forty-five unless there is no other alternative. In this case, there was not. Mike had fractured his left hip years earlier, and it had deteriorated to the point where he was suffering excruciating pain.

Dr. Lesher opened the hip, cut off the head of the femur, and reamed diseased bone and cartilage from the acetabular area, while Dr. Singletary assisted. I stood to the side and watched; my primary role that day, I thought, was to make sure the nurses handed Dr. Lesher the right instruments. The case went well until Lesher started having trouble finding the correct degree of anteversion, the angle at which the cup should sit in the hip. He used a positioning instrument with a round ball that fits into the cup.

To align the positioner, the surgeon places the patient flat on his back and the operating table in a horizontal position. He then moves the handle to a 45-degree angle from the midline of the body, looking at the patient from above. Viewing the patient from the side, the positioner insures that the cup is tilted slightly upward in the hip socket. If the cup is wrongly angled in either plane, the two components of the artificial hip will probably dislocate. Thus, positioning is a crucial part of a total hip procedure, and a major cause of disaster. Only by doing it often can a surgeon become adept at this technique. He must also learn to do it quickly, for once the methylmethacrylate cement is mixed, he has about five minutes before it hardens. During this time he must work the cement into the reamed-out acetabulum, insert the acetabular cup, position it at the correct angle, press the cup into place to create a good bond, and remove excess cement with a curette. If the cement sets before all this is done, the entire procedure must be repeated, with the added problem of removing the cement.

On this particular day, as Dr. Lesher struggled to position the cup, he asked me whether the angle was correct. I said, no, and tried to explain how to orient the cup positioner.

"The cement is getting hard," he said. "Would you please do it for me?"

I took the instrument, moved it to the correct angle, and

positioned the cup in the acetabulum. Lesher then reamed the femoral canal and inserted the prosthesis for a trial reduction. He put the patient's leg through a range of motion. The results looked good, so good in fact that the new prosthesis corrected a two-inch shortening the patient had in the right leg. Lesher cemented the femoral prosthesis in place, I positioned it, and we both tested it, again with success.

Now came the task of rewiring the greater trochanter and its attachment, the gluteus minimus muscle that holds the femur in the hip socket. At the beginning of the procedure, Lesher had removed the greater trochanter with a Gigli saw and moved it aside to allow better access to the acetabulum. Now he had to rewire the greater trochanter even tighter to the femur, to re-establish tension in the muscles so they could act like a large rubber band and hold the hip joint together.

"Bill," he said, "you've done this before. Give me a hand with this rewiring."

"Sure, Doctor." By now I had learned that "give me a hand" means "do it."

I doubled an eighteen-gauge wire and, after fumbling a while, managed to insert it through a hole Lesher had drilled through the femoral shaft. Four wire ends protruded from the bone. These I inserted through two holes Lesher had drilled in the greater trochanter. He finished the job with a Kirschner wire tractor, which tightens the wire into a neat twist. As he pulled and turned the instrument, I thought to myself, "Don't be so heavy-handed. You'll pop the wire and we'll end up doing the job over again." But Lesher finished without mishap and the final result looked like a neatly wrapped package. The proper tension had been restored to the gluteus minimus muscle, and the greater trochanter was back where it belonged. Lesher closed up the hip incision, and brought the case to a close. The next day I visited Mike, who was feeling little pain, considering what he had been through.

The true test of surgical success, however, came about a year later when he was knocked down by a tractor, dragged about eight feet, and did not hurt his hip.

A few months later, I scrubbed in on another case that brought my level of participation suddenly to new heights. Prior to the case I had shown Drs. John Perth and Marshall Brokaw, I will call them, a new device, a compression hip screw, which is used to repair fractures of the femoral neck. This three-part device consists of a plate that runs along the femur, a lag screw that is embedded in the femoral head, and a small screw that draws the lag screw (and the femoral head) toward the plate. This creates compression and unites the fracture until it can grow together.

Dr. Perth decided, soon after I showed him the product, to try it on a patient with a fractured hip. The morning of the case he called and invited me to attend. The surgery was scheduled at three in the afternoon. When I arrived in the OR, I found only an anesthesiologist, a scrub nurse, and Dr. Perth. A circulating nurse came in and out, but she was absent for the most part. Dr. Perth made a seven-inch incision and inserted three guidewires to determine which angle the hip screw should take. The angle must be exact or the hip screw and plate will not fit flush against the femur. After inserting the wires, Dr. Perth ordered X rays, decided which angle to use, and pulled the other two guidewires out. Perth then took a nail starter, a small drill that fits over the wire, and drilled a hole the exact shape of the lag screw, which had different diameters at different points. He inserted the screw and, with a clockwise motion, cranked it into the femoral neck and head with a special socket wrench. After a few minutes, he tried to slide the angled tube of the compression plate over the lag screw by twisting it clockwise. It would not fit. He tried it counterclockwise. No luck. He fumbled a while longer, and I could sense his frustration mounting as the minutes ticked away.

Finally he looked at the scrub nurse and said, "The hell with this. I'm going to put a Smith-Peterson plate in this guy."

This is an entirely different procedure, so I said, "Doctor, wait a minute, it's not that hard."

My cajoling was apparently adding to his frustration. He continued to fume and suddenly picked up an instrument—I never saw what—and threw it across the room.

"Dr. Perth," I said, "the lag screw is in, and we'll get the plate in too."

But Perth was not to be consoled. "*You* put the fuckin' thing in," he bellowed and strode into the next room and started looking at X rays on the viewbox.

The moment I realized that he had turned the entire case over to me and left me operating solo, I felt shocked. Then fear set in. I had stepped into cases before, but never alone, with only an anesthesiologist and scrub nurse at my side.

"What if I screw it up, instead of in?" I thought in panic, for I had never done a compression plate before. Then I remembered: "I've done hips. I've done knees. Why not this?" My fear vanished.

Thus, for the next twenty-five minutes I worked alone on the patient. I began by turning the compression plate onto the lag screw, not with the doctor's quick turns, but with the slow movements a safecracker would use while searching out numbers of the dial of a safe. I rotated the plate in a clockwise direction with a slight pressure until I felt the threads on the plate engage the threads on the lag screw. When I felt the comforting click that told me the plate had slid on, I said to myself, "Thank God."

To the scrub nurse I said, "Hand me the compression screw," the third part of the implant, which tightened the plate to the lag screw. I had always told surgeons they could actually feel the bone fragments compressing when they turned the screw. Now it was my turn with the surgical screwdriver, and I could feel the compression pull the fractured femoral head back into the main part of the bone. As soon as the tension felt right—a carpenter would know what I mean—I stopped turning and asked for an orthotome drill. While I worked, the scrub nurse kept looking at me without uttering a word. But the question flickered in her eyes: "What's going on here?"

The anesthesiologist, who was the only physician in the room, sat at the patient's head, equally and stonily silent. I drilled four holes for bone screws to hold the compression plate snug against the femur and crooked my left index finger around the femur to be sure I had drilled clear through. Just as I decided to use inch-and-a-quarter screws, Perth walked back into the room, never even glancing at what I had done.

"How're we doing?"

"I'm ready to put the bone screws in and we'll be finished."

"Oh, okay."

I moved aside to make room for him, but he showed no interest in the task. As soon as I finished with the fourth screw, he said, "All right, let's close up and get the hell out of here."

Perth stitched while I cut sutures. Then a technician from the X-ray department came and took two X rays of the hip. Perth thanked me for helping out, and that was the end of the case. But it was not the end of my reflections about it. I had never seen a surgeon become so incensed by a procedure not going his way.

That day it seemed as if his hands would not work for him. He was all thumbs. He had always struck me as the type of orthopedic surgeon who, if something did not fit, would hit it with a hammer and *make* it fit. He had no finesse.

After Perth left, I stayed in greens and waited for Dr. Brokaw to arrive for the next case. He planned to install the same compression hip screw as Perth and I had just done. When Brokaw arrived he asked, "How did the case go with John?" I shrugged my shoulders.

"What do you mean?" he asked.

"John couldn't get the plate on, and he walked out of the room on me, so I buttoned it in."

"Oh, is everything okay with the patient?"

I replied that the patient was fine, but I wondered why Brokaw did not ask for more details. Perhaps, I decided, he considered it par for the course. In terms of body language, however, I must admit that Brokaw did a double-take when I told him that Perth had stormed out of the operating room and left me alone.

Brokaw then turned to the case at hand, and asked me to talk through the procedure for him. As I described each step (from my head and not from Xeroxed instructions) he carried it out as easily as 1, 2, 3, even though he, too, had never done a compression plate before. In thirty minutes we were finished, skin to skin, meaning initial incision to closure. It was a tribute to Brokaw's excellence as a trauma surgeon, for the operation ordinarily takes more than an hour, and the Perth rendition took an hour and a half.

By 1974 I was attending all the total hip surgery at several hospitals, partly, though not entirely, because I loaned them the instruments they needed. I also did a considerable amount of surgery at another hospital, which owned its own instruments for Charnley total hip procedures but whose surgeons invited me nonetheless.

Around that time Dr. Walter DeYoung, as I will call him, was planning his first total hip replacement. He called several weeks ahead to ask what kind of hip I recommended. He also wanted to see appropriate movies of the procedure so he could learn it as well as possible beforehand. On my advice, he decided to use the T-28 (trapezoidal 28-millimeter head) total hip prosthesis manufactured by my company. This hip prosthesis resembles the one used in the Charnley procedure except that the neck and shaft of the femoral component are trapezoidal and the head is larger.

The instruments for installing this hip, however, are quite different from those used in the Charnley procedures Dr. DeYoung had attended. It was also the first total hip procedure where Dr. DeYoung was in charge and not assisting somebody else.

On the morning of the operation, I brought the necessary instruments. En route to the operating room, I saw the patient lying on a wheeled stretcher outside the operating room. I stopped to chat, and he told me he was having both hips "done"—this was the first of two operations—so he could dance at his daughter's wedding. Within ten minutes he was in the operating room, anesthetized and blissfully unaware of the song and dance that went on that day. From start to finish, the case was like a scene from *M*A*S*H.*

Dr. Walter DeYoung, a quiet man in his fifties, was assisted by Dr. Paul Christine, I will call him, while another salesman and I observed. As the procedure started, Dr. DeYoung put X rays on the viewer, which served as Christine's cue to begin telling DeYoung how to proceed with the surgery. DeYoung said, "I've got it pretty well planned, Paul." Christine was well aware that this was DeYoung's first total hip.

DeYoung's initial incision, a curvilinear cut, measured about ten inches. The patient was propped on his side with rolled-up sheets to keep him from falling. The affected hip faced upward. As DeYoung opened the subcutaneous tissue, the blood-suctioning equipment kept getting clogged with debris. "Nurse, the suctioning is not working properly," DeYoung kept saying. But the circulating nurse was not checking the bottle of blood on the floor or squeezing the tube to keep it flowing free. She was too busy sitting in the corner taking an inventory in one of the closets that lined the operating-room wall.

Meanwhile, the anesthesiologist wore his mask over his mouth but not his nose. DeYoung turned to him and said, "Will you please pick up your mask?"

"Oh, yeah, yeah, Doctor."

A few minutes later, the mask was down again. DeYoung, who was being very cautious about sterility violations, reminded the anesthesiologist about his mask again. After the fourth request, he finally complied, under protest: "I have to wear a mask all day. You're here for only one case."

DeYoung, in the meantime, removed the greater trochanter, exposed the femoral head, and dislocated the hip. He was now ready to ream the acetabulum. He used a Mira power reamer I had loaned the hospital, along with instruments for the T-28 total hip. (My boss expected me to get a purchase order for a reamer after the case.) This instrument is a mushroom-shaped drill with a sharp blade running transsectionally through the middle. DeYoung attached the reamer to a Hall II air driver which operates up to 20,000 rpm, and began reaming cartilage and soft-tissue debris from the acetabulum. Paul Christine was holding Hohmann retractors as DeYoung reamed, and reamed, and reamed. Something did not seem right, and I asked to see the reamer. He raised it up, but it showed no debris, bone, or anything else. Instead of reaming, the instrument was bouncing up and down in the patient like a broken washing machine: BABOOM, BABOOM, BABOOM.

"Lean on it. Bear down on it, Doctor," I said.

"I don't know how hard to lean on it," he said.

"Let me show you."

He moved to the right, and I took the reamer, pressed on it hard, and immediately felt the RHRRRRRRRRRR vibrate in the handle and up through my arms as the reamer grabbed onto the bone.

"Now we've got it, Doctor." When I lifted the reamer out of the socket, it was covered with blood and bone.

"Now you try it," I said. He put it back into the hip socket. BABOOM, BABOOM, BABOOM.

"Here, let me do it again."

And again it went RHRRRRRRRRRR.

I continued reaming the acetabulum, and later wished I had done the whole job, because the reamer was scratched so badly that my boss deducted more than a hundred dollars from my paycheck to cover it. The instrument was scratched because DeYoung had been reaming one of the steel Hohmann retractors instead of the acetabulum!

Meanwhile, Dr. Paul Christine had criticized us continuously for reaming the acetabulum bed from the wrong angle. Christine was so overbearing, telling DeYoung how to do the case and trying, I felt, to take it over completely, that I sided with DeYoung.

"Just do your own thing," I told him. "It's your case, so don't let anybody else talk you into anything."

I think he appreciated my support, because he said "Thanks, Bill," very quietly.

At this point Christine mixed the methylmethacrylate bone cement and handed it to DeYoung, who shaped it like a hamburger patty and pressed it into the acetabulum. He took the cup and the positioning instrument. "Bill, what do you think? Am I all right? Put your hands on mine and make sure I'm in the right position." For five minutes, I placed my hands over his and helped him position the acetabular cup. My hands, in effect, told his what to do. I assume he wanted to know, in the future, how to do it himself.

Christine, still the professor, said, "That looks good, Walt. I like the way you're doing that." I had the feeling that if DeYoung had walked away from the table for a minute to look at X rays, Christine would have stepped in and started cutting. But De-Young never gave Christine a chance. He reamed out the femur, drilled holes for reattaching the greater trochanter, tested the leg for range of motion. I guided his hands when he cemented the prosthesis in the shaft, and helped him position it. I rewired the greater trochanter, and DeYoung and I finished up the case.

The other salesman and I went to the coffee shop afterward, and when we were seated, he said, "You gotta be kidding me!"

"What do you mean?"

"You know, MacKay, I've known you for a couple of years. I knew you were doing a lot of surgery, because that's the only way you could get the amount of business you have. But I never would have believed you were doing surgery to this extent. These guys don't shit unless they ask you!"

About a month later, the patient returned to the hospital for a second hip operation, and I scrubbed in on the case. But I never learned whether he danced again. This man suffered from arthritis, a reason many hips are replaced. Arthritis is a disease that, in some of its dozens of forms, attacks the joints, causes stiffening, loss of motion, and excruciating pain. In many cases, the femoral head is eroded and the cartilage, which acts as a sponge or buffer between the bones and keeps them from grinding against one another, is eaten away. In other cases the hip joint must be replaced because the femoral head is necrotic— dead—and has lost its blood supply. Hip joints are also replaced because a prosthesis has failed, because the patient has poor bone stock in the hip region, or because he cannot be treated by other means.

After rewiring the greater trochanter of the man who wanted to dance again, I had a chance to demonstrate an improvement I had made in that technique. The opportunity came when Dr. Marshall Brokaw called me while I was attending the annual meeting of the American Academy of Orthopedic Surgeons in Dallas, Texas. Brokaw tracked me down by telephone and asked if I could return a few days early to attend a total hip case. I agreed to return in time for the operation. Dr. Perth was assisting. As I entered the OR, the scrub nurse asked if I would help her because she was not totally familiar with the instrumentation for the Charnley procedure. I agreed to pass instruments to the doctor and essentially became the scrub nurse in the case. The operation progressed normally until Brokaw had trouble determining the depth and position of the reamer. He asked for help, and I reamed the acetabulum.

When it was time to drill holes for the wires used to reattach the greater trochanter, I suggested a faster way of doing it. I had been working for many evenings on a new wiring technique on the cadaver bones in my garage. Brokaw agreed to my idea because he was always interested in saving time. The old Charnley wiring technique was extremely difficult and time-consuming. It required more wire than my idea, and more drill holes in the femur. And the old technique placed considerable strain on the wire when the surgeon tightened it down. My technique, on the other hand, required less wire, one less hole in the femur, and less tension on the wire. That meant it would not stretch or be as likely to break later on. Although the bone grows back in most cases, it does not always. Meanwhile, the muscles in that region pull against that wire and create enormous stress. Orthopedic journals report that the wires used in the Charnley total hip procedure can break, sometimes making further surgery necessary. My technique greatly reduced that danger, simplified the case, and reduced operative time by about fifteen minutes. This was the first, but not last, application of my wiring idea. Dr. Brokaw later discussed the technique at an orthopedic conference. Several surgeons asked about the technique and showed no surprise at my having developed and applied it.

In fact, ever since my first total hip case with Tom Merriman almost two years earlier, many doctors in the Long Island area knew about my participation in surgery. After that operation, Dr.

Merriman had invited me to an orthopedic conference where the surgeons who attended seemed totally aware of my role in that procedure. From then on, they began increasingly to consult me about many matters, from new prostheses to the surgical problems in implanting them. In many instances, they asked for help in preparing their cases. Other times, they asked for help in correcting their errors. Unfortunately, the latter instances were all too frequent.

SIX

THE
TOTAL SALE

A colleague in the orthopedic business once called me the best salesman he had ever met. Since he was a competitor and a good salesman himself, I took his statement to be high praise. Selling is a difficult, cut-throat business. The key is to sell your company's product. If you fail, financially speaking, you are dead. So I sold as hard as I could, and sometimes I made friends and sometimes I made enemies. But it was all part of the game.

My selling technique was based on two premises. First, I would give the best possible service to the doctors. Secondly, I had to know more about implants than anyone else—including the competition and, sometimes, the surgeons themselves. With time and experience, my techniques evolved into the *total sale*. It worked best on a Saturday morning when I attended a hospital's monthly orthopedic conference where doctors would meet to discuss recent cases of interest. I was specifically interested in attending the meetings at the smaller private hospitals, for they were my biggest accounts. The large teaching hospitals also held orthopedic conferences, but I was less interested in these because they dealt mainly with trauma cases. In my scale of priorities, the opportunity to sell an artificial hip costing $350 outranked a $1.85 pin used in the average trauma case.

A typical conference would take place in the hospital cafeteria around two large conference tables placed at right angles. At the head sat the Chief of Orthopedics. Behind him a multiple viewbox stood ready to display X rays. By 8:30 A.M., fifteen to twenty surgeons (many have privileges in several hospitals) arrived bearing X rays and case notes. The meeting usually began calmly enough. Dr. X announced that he wanted to present a case and snapped an X ray on the viewer.

"This is a twenty-nine-year-old female Caucasian and, as you can see here, she has fractured her clavicle. Because of the nature of the fracture, I decided to pin it rather than put it in a brace."

He then produced another X ray: "Here we are three months post-op, and you can see that . . ." The interesting thing is that these doctors invariably presented their successful cases, but not their disasters.

The next cases would cut closer to the bone. The battle lines between conservative surgeons, who wanted to cast, and the nonconservative, who wanted to cut, would be clearly drawn. Dr. Carl Gilford, for example, once presented a case of a sixteen-year-old girl with a slipped wrist epiphysis, a plate of bone at the lower end of the radius or forearm. Historically, this type of injury has been treated conservatively by putting it in a cast. But Gilford preferred to install a pin surgically, and showed X rays of the procedure. Charlie Singletary stood up and said, "Carl, I don't know how you can sleep with yourself at night! Why did you pin this epiphysis?"

"I decided to because . . ."

"Can you show me in the literature where this has been done?"

"They're treating this problem surgically in Germany. They've found that . . ."

Then the meeting took a not-unexpected twist. Dr. Walter DeYoung broke in: "You know, Charlie [speaking to Singletary], I've been looking at the emergency-room log from last month, and I want to know how you are getting all those patients."

"They come in and ask for me," Singletary replied.

"Charlie, why are they asking for *you*?"

"Well, you know, I've got a reputation . . ."

"Charlie, you've been here three stinking years. How much of a reputation can you have? What the hell is happening in the emergency room?"

(The answer was that Singletary had cultivated the nurses to the point where they called him instead of the doctor on the roster to attend to a case and, in the process, acquire a new patient.)

Then Tom Merriman chimed in: "Yeah, you know, it's funny. My emergency-room patients have fallen off." From the back of the room, another voice:

"Hey, mine have too!"

Somebody asked Singletary's partner: "Norman, how come you're always in the emergency room? Every time I go there, day or night, you guys are always there!"

Tom Merriman finally restored order, and several more sets of X rays went up on the viewer.

At last it was my turn, as Dr. DeYoung announced, "I've asked Bill MacKay here today to show us a film on the Marmor total knee. Bill, do you want to go ahead now?"

"Sure, Dr. DeYoung." I dimmed the lights, turned on the projector, and ran a twenty-minute movie with sound track. When the lights flicked back on, I waited for the usual questions about the clinical background on the knee. This was my cue to cite the latest article in the *Journal of Bone and Joint Surgery*. At that point I would take the knee prosthesis, which I had polished to a high sheen, and move the components against one another, showing the doctors the range of motion and rotation features. Then I would place the knee prosthesis, along with several dozen instruments I sold for implanting it, on boards covered with red velvet where, like jewels, they beckoned the doctors to look, touch, buy. . . .

I would try to hold my audience in thrall as long as possible, since it meant twenty or so fewer doctors I would have to chase afterward in their offices.

This I did in a variety of ways. One of the most effective was to engage in debate with one of the doctors. I recall one occasion when a doctor remarked that a specific type hip was easiest to implant because the greater trochanter did not have to be removed, and the implant more closely resembled the natural hip. He added that these hips were made of Vitallium, a cobalt-chromium alloy that is more inert than surgical steel. When he finished I asked, "Are you familiar with the recent report in the *Journal of Bone and Joint Surgery* on the repeated breakage of this type of stem?"

"No, I'm not."

"Doctor, are you familiar with reports by two doctors in Massachusetts on the reactions of tissue to Vitallium?"

No answer.

"Are you aware of reports on the fatigue factor of Vitallium as opposed to steel?"

"Well, you know . . ."

"Doctor, Vitallium is a brittle metal, whereas steel is stronger and more ductile. Would you agree that ultimately weight must be transmitted to the heel?"

"Yes, I agree with that."

"Fine. A Charnley hip is placed in the patient medially to place stress on the inner side of the femur. When you put in the type you are using, the placement is not as medial, and stress is transferred to the stem of the prosthesis; do you agree?"

"Well, yes."

"Then can you explain to me, if Vitallium is not as strong as steel, how can we expect the prosthesis, placed in a way that produces more strain, to last?"

All the while, the doctor sat staring at a piece of paper and tapping it with the eraser, then the point, of his pencil. My object was to overwhelm him with expertise. My debates usually succeeded because I did my homework.

When the debates ended my real selling would begin. Several doctors interested in implanting a total knee would start asking me about it. This would be my opportunity to do business, for even though I was selling a knee that day, I also would have a whole bag of other instruments along. "Did you see this new nail guide?" I would say. "It helps you get the right angle on a Jewett nailing."

"That really looks good," a doctor would say.

"Do you want me to send you one?"

He would nod, my cue to mail it to his office and bill him.

Another doctor would come up to me:

"Hi, Bill, how are you doing?"

"Good, Charlie. Did you see this new broach that's come out? The idea is that you can take off more bone medially, so you don't have to rasp as much."

"Hey, that looks pretty good."

"Charlie, do you want one of these?"

"Well, I don't want to buy it."

"Okay, tell you what. Write me a prescription now and I'll have the OR supervisor order it for you."

He would then write out a prescription. The following Monday morning, I would go to the OR supervisor and say, "I saw Dr. Singletary on Saturday, and showed him a new broach that will reduce operative time. He wants one."

"Well, have Dr. Singletary write me a note telling me he wants one."

I would then produce the prescription from my pocket.

"Fine, Bill, I'll order it this week."

There was another technique: going first to the hospital administrator who makes the final decision. "I was talking to some doctors," I would say, "and they would really love to have this new hip system."

"How much is it, Bill?"

"It's going to run you about seven thousand. They really want it because it's a good system."

"Why don't you speak to the OR supervisor and have her put in a requisition?"

Next I would chat with the directress of nursing and tell her that I'd already spoken to the hospital administrator. By the time I saw the OR supervisor, the next level down, she was inclined to approve the order because she knew there would be no static higher up.

One of the simplest methods was to appeal to the doctors' intelligence by posing a suggestion in the form of a question. In surgery I never said, "Doctor, you should do it his way." I would say, "Doctor, what do you think about doing this?" or "Some of the other surgeons think this is the method of choice." Even when my hands, and not the surgeon's, were inside a patient, I would say "we," thereby taking command in deed, but never in words. The "we technique" worked well on everybody, but was especially effective on surgeons, who are not known to be shrinking violets, because it allowed them to take responsibility for the idea. If it succeeded, they could take credit. If it failed, they could blame me.

I also specialized in learning first names of doctors, their wives, children, plus their hobbies, favorite sports, and even on occasion, the characteristics of their dogs and cats. I would painstakingly compile this information and enter it on a card file. When I called on a doctor, I could then relate to him on many levels. This would put him in a positive frame of mind, and build a bridge to what I wanted to talk about: the product I was selling.

I learned about the operating-room supervisors as well. During a sales call I might discover it was a supervisor's day off. Most salesmen at this point would say, "Well, I'll catch her next week." I would stay and ask the nurse on duty, "By the way, when is Louise's birthday?"

"I think it's January sixth. Why do you want to know?"

"Our company likes to send a birthday card to the supervisors."

Actually, the company did not care about her birthday. I sent the card, along with a red silk rose for her desk.

Flexibility is another hallmark of the successful salesman. When I changed companies, I was suddenly selling prosthetic hips and knees that, only a month earlier, I had been competing against. When selling my original company's line I argued at an orthopedic conference that my rival's Cathcart artificial hip, with its egg-shaped—instead of round—femoral component, would create more friction in the joint than my company's spherical prosthesis. At the time I contended that the less the friction, the less the wear on the acetabulum. Then, when I started selling the other line, I suddenly recognized the advantages of the Cathcart, and I emphasized that the friction caused by the Cathcart elliptical prosthesis was, in fact, beneficial, for it helped pump synovial fluid to lubricate the hip socket.

But the most intricate maneuvers in a salesman's repertoire are directed at (perhaps I should say against) other salesmen. Competition was so intense it called for an ongoing attack on a daily basis. A good salesman always uses psychological warfare against his competitors. One of my main strategies was to make a point of running into one of my competitors in the lobby of his biggest hospital account.

"Hi, how are you?" I would say.

"Uh, okay, Bill."

"Let's grab a cup of coffee."

In the luncheonette of that hospital, I would ask about his wife, kids, then talk about baseball or whatever else interested him. Then I would say, "By the way, have you had this account a long time?"

"I've had it fourteen months."

"What would happen if you lost this account?"

"I can't lose this. I'm solid here."

I would look at him and say, "I really don't want to upset you. You look like a nice guy and I know you've got a family and everything, but I just want you to know *I'm taking this account away from you.*"

He would look at me in disbelief, then laugh it off and say, "Sure, Bill, you just do that!" But the next day the chances were good that he would start overreacting by spending extra time with all the doctors and nurses on his calling list and make a general nuisance of himself. He would probably tell people I was trying to steal his account. In the process he would become my best advertisement. Then I would visit the same offices, introduce myself, and tell the doctors I would be servicing the account for my company. "I realize you are a busy man," I would say, "but if there's anything I can do to help you, just let me know. I'll leave my card with you." I would be polite without even an inkling of pressure. The person I had just met would probably think, "Gee, he isn't such a bad guy. The other salesman said he was a pushy SOB." And immediately a credibility question would form about the other salesman.

Next I would look for the easiest pieces of the action to take from the other salesman: slings, knee braces, and other soft goods. As I took these, he would overreact even more, trying to save his business. The more he overreacted, the more he would lose. Before long, I would have the whole hospital and he would be on the outside looking in. As a follow-up, I would make sure I ran into him again. "Jack," I would say, "that was really too easy. Now I'm going to take such-and-such hospital from you."

This technique didn't win any popularity contests. But most salesmen were so lacking in energy and drive that I hardly needed to wage such strenuous campaigns to take business from them. Few of my competitors ever attended a Saturday-morning orthopedic conference despite the richness of sales opportunities. They played golf on Saturday instead. I played golf during the week and attended conferences on Saturday. Even when other salesmen did attend conferences, they usually left as soon as they ended, just when my selling began. Seldom did a competitor contribute anything during the meeting as I did. I could elaborate on the different types of appliances the doctors could use for a specific problem illuminated on the viewbox. Other salesmen did not because they did not do their homework and were afraid they would be asked a question they could not answer. So while they played in their spare time, I was out working. My payoff came in the form of ever-increasing, record-breaking sales.

SEVEN

THE CASE OF
THE UNHINGED
KNEE

An unusual case in August 1974 illustrates how I was drawn—by the efforts of many people and not just of a single doctor—into covering up a surgical error. Early that month, Dr. Carl Gilford told me he wanted to implant a hinge knee in an elderly man with rheumatoid arthritis. Artificial knees were extremely experimental at this point, and of all the types of total knees available, hinge knees were perhaps the least reliable. But my function was to sell, not question, them. So I recommended that he try a new Guepar-type hinge knee. Dr. Gilford told me to order the knee and scheduled the case a week hence. I did not attend the procedure because I had other things to do that day. Nor do I recall that Dr. Gilford asked me to attend.

About a week or so after the case, a problem arose. To understand it requires an explanation of how a hinge knee differs from a total knee. The latter is a ball-and-cup device, with the ball made of metal and the cup an ultra-high-molecular-weight plastic. The hinge knee, made entirely of metal, works essentially like a door hinge, with the interlocking femoral and tibial parts held together by a pin with a diameter about the size of a dime.

The operation requires a minimum of bone removal and

only a few special instruments, in contrast to the templates, saws, and chisels of the total knee procedure. Installing the hinge knee is merely a matter of cutting off the condyles on the femur horizontally and similarly planing the top of the tibia. The surgeon then takes a rasp (or broach) and reams a hole in the medullary canal of the femur. He does the same in the medullary canal of the tibia, puts cement in each canal, and inserts the two components, each of which has a spike on the end. It is a straightforward, uncomplicated procedure, provided the surgeon does it right.

About a week after the case, Dr. Gilford called. "Bill, I want you to come over to my office right away to look at an X ray," When I arrived, he held up a film that showed the hinge pin moving out of position.

"I don't know what's wrong," he said.

"Did you put the C-washer on?" I asked. (This is a small ring that locks the hinge pin in place.)

"Sure, sure. And then I put the pin in lateral to medial."

"Carl, wait a minute, the instructions say to put the prosthesis in *medial* to *lateral,*" meaning from inside to outside the knee.

"Oh, I must have put it in backwards!" He pondered this discovery several minutes, then said, "Why don't you call the manufacturer, Bill, and ask what we can do."

I picked up the phone in his office and called the engineering department at my company. I reached a biomechanical engineer who took fifteen minutes to figure out what I was talking about. When he finally grasped the situation—that Dr. Gilford had inserted a hinge pin from the wrong side—he reminded me that a sheet of instructions comes with every Guepar knee.

"The surgeon says they weren't in the box," I said.

"Yes they were," he said.

We spent ten more minutes arguing over that. The instructions, he lectured, state very clearly that the hinge-pin mechanism *must* be inserted from the medial side to the lateral side. "If it is done backward, there is no locking mechanism to hold the hinge pin in place. In other words, he's going to have to redo the knee."

I relayed the news to Gilford, and recommended that he insert a new hinge pin, since the one that was migrating around in the patient's knee was probably a bit worn. Gilford agreed to reoperate, but not right away. He was about to leave for Mexico for a week's vacation, he said, and the patient would have to wait until his return. I told him that it was his decision, but I thought he should first hospitalize the patient, make two small incisions on either side of his knee, and switch the pin around. In fact, the case could have been booked as an emergency the following morning, when it would have taken precedence over every other scheduled procedure.

I did not approve of the way Gilford proposed to solve the problem, nor did I admire his carelessness in creating it. I had delivered the knee to him several days before the case, and he had had the time to find out whether the instructions were inside the box. If they were missing, as he claimed, he could have obtained another set, or read about the procedure in the medical literature, or in some way prepared himself. Now we had a crisis on our hands.

The next day I received a message at my office to call Janet Geffen, as I will call the directress of nursing at the hospital where the surgery was scheduled.

"Hi, Janet. How are you?" I said.

"I'm very concerned about this hinge knee that Dr. Gilford just did. The thing's coming apart, and I'm afraid of a malpractice suit. What do you think we should do?"

"Look, Janet, I've already called our engineering department and they're sending a new pin. I'm going to get the purchase order from the operating-room supervisor today. As soon as the pin arrives, we'll take care of it."

"All right. Do you feel you have this under control?"

I assured her that I did, and she told me that Jerry Vargas, the name I will give to the hospital administrator, and Dr. Nicholas Coffield, my name for the Chief of Surgery, wanted to speak to me.

About one o'clock the next day, while I was calling on some doctors, I received a message from my office to call Dr. Coffield. He was not in his office. I dialed the hospital number and asked the switchboard to page Dr. Coffield.

"This is Bill MacKay returning your call."

"Yes, yes. I wanted to speak to you about the patient Dr. Gilford did the other day. What's the situation?" I told him the hinge pin was in backward and that Dr. Gilford would have to operate again to replace it.

"Why weren't you in on the case?"

"Because, number one, Dr. Gilford didn't ask me to be there. Number two, the instructions in the package clearly state that the hinge pin must be inserted medial to lateral. It was done exactly the opposite, lateral to medial, which is why you have this problem. So don't lay it on my shoulders."

"Let's not jump all over one another's backs. I'm not trying to blame you or anybody else, I just want to rectify this situation. Otherwise this man is going to sue. What happens if he goes to another doctor and he finds a hinge pin migrating around in the knee?"

"Doctor, what are you asking me?"

"I'm asking what you think we should do."

"Personally, if it were my patient, I would put him in plaster up to his hips."

"Why do that?"

"Because, if you put an Ace bandage on him, the hinge pin will begin to annoy him and sooner or later he will pick up the phone and call another orthopedic surgeon. He'll X-ray the knee and see that the pin has dislodged. And then he is going to sue the balls off you people."

I explained to Dr. Coffield that if they put the patient in plaster to the point of immobilizing him, he might be very content to lie at home in bed rather than venture forth to see another orthopedist. Nor would he be as likely to seek help because he would not feel as much pain. "As soon as Dr. Gilford returns from Mexico you can reoperate, and no one will ever know the pin was put in backward."

Actually there was a sound medical reason for putting the patient in plaster. Immobilizing him reduced the possibility of the hinge pin migrating all the way out and causing the knee to dislocate. If the knee had dislocated, the prosthesis could have broken through the skin. Or it could have severed an artery. Coffield liked my idea.

"I'm going to tell Gilford to put him in plaster up to his neck! But when he returns, I want you to be at that procedure and make sure it goes right."

"Dr. Coffield, I'll be more than happy to be present for the surgery; however, I'm sure Dr. Gilford will have an assistant."

Up to this point, I had scrubbed at several of Dr. Gilford's total hip cases because he wanted to maintain sterility in the operating room. But I had never touched any of his patients.

Coffield was insistent: "Should I bring in an outside consultant?"

I said no.

"Well, I want you in the case," he said. "I know you scrub in on all the total hips, and I want to make sure the knee is done properly this time."

I agreed, but felt very concerned when I hung up. Bringing in an outside consultant to look over Gilford's shoulder was, in effect, a disciplinary measure and an embarrassment. I called Dr. Gilford just as he was leaving for the airport, and told him what Coffield had said about bringing in another doctor as a consultant. He thanked me for the warning, and said he wanted me to be there for the case.

As soon as Dr. Gilford returned from vacation, I received a phone call from Jerry Vargas, the hospital administrator. He said, "I have been talking to Dr. Coffield and Janet Geffen, and we have to reoperate on a patient with a hinge knee. I want you to be goddam sure the thing goes in right this time."

"It's really a simple case," I told him. "All they have to do is make two incisions on each side of the knee, slide the old hinge pin out and the new one in, in the right direction, of course. I'll be glad to give the surgeons any technical advice they want."

"Let's be candid with one another," he said. "I'm afraid of a malpractice suit in this case. Just be there, and do whatever needs to be done."

The mandate was clear. I said, as I had to Dr. Coffield: "Yes, sir."

I was worried by these calls insisting that I attend the hinge-pin replacement. Unlike other invitations I had received from surgeons to scrub in on their cases, these were marching orders, not a request. I could have refused, but I felt I could be helpful to the patient and, frankly, I was concerned about losing business at the hospital, which was one of my major accounts. It seemed obvious that if I refused the demands of the hospital administrator and the chief of surgery, I was not going to sell equipment there much longer. They had said nothing specific, but the veiled threat was unmistakable: If you do not take care of our needs, whatever they may be, there are other salesmen who will.

Several days later I ran into Dr. Coffield in the hospital's lobby. Would I be there for the knee procedure? I assured him I would, and asked who the attending surgeon would be. "Benjamin Frolich," he told me.

"What if Frolich [as I call him] tries to get in on the act?" I asked.

"Just tell Frolich to get the hell out of the room."

On the day of surgery, I went to the operating room, not Number 4, where most of the orthopedics are done, but another room.

The patient was brought in and put on the table. Gilford stood on the left side nearest to the knee we were repairing. Frolich stood to the patient's right, and I stood at the foot of the table, where I could not see anything because of draping.

The knee was bent into a 90-degree angle and Gilford announced how he planned to do the procedure. Then Frolich said, "I think we ought to do it this way." Then my turn: "Let's make two percutaneous incisions, slide the old pin out, insert the new pin medial to lateral, and get the hell out of here." Gilford said, "Fine," and made a two-inch incision on either side of the knee. He asked the scrub nurse for a pair of Kelly clamps, which look like very finely pointed pliers. He reached through the inner (medial) side of the knee and removed a small lock washer that had been flattened out and obviously had not done its job. Gilford suggested sliding in the new pin as we removed the old, so that the knee components would not come apart.

Dr. Frolich, who had been holding retractors, made a move that suggested he was getting ready to help replace the pin. Gilford interrupted him: "No, no, let Bill help me with this." Dr. Frolich continued to stand in front of me and block my view as well as my access to the knee. Gilford asked me again for help with the pin, and I said, "Doctor, I can't give you a hand. Dr. Frolich is right in front of me." With that, Dr. Gilford looked at him and said, "Ben, would you get out of the way and let Bill in here?"

After changing places with Dr. Frolich, I put my thumb inside the patient's knee and pushed in the new pin while Dr. Gilford simultaneously guided out the old pin from the patient's left side. I pushed it through medial to lateral, while Gilford attached a new plastic C-washer on the lateral side of the knee, and snapped it together. The new pin fit beautifully. There were no complications inserting it, and the entire case took about thirty minutes. I left before Gilford sewed up the two incisions.

In the doctor's lounge, as I changed back to street clothes, I thought, "What a bunch of hypocrites these people are. Everybody's playing hospital politics."

It troubled me even more that I had participated in covering up a surgical error. It is true that I was ordered to participate, but

I also consented. As for my suggestion to cover the patient with plaster, at the time it seemed more like an attempt to rectify than conceal an error, and since Dr. Gilford had elected to go on vacation, it was a question of buying time until he returned. In the final analysis, I was the one who not only helped cover up but suggested *how* the cover-up should be accomplished. And I did not like the feeling of being involved in such a fashion. It was wrong.

EIGHT
VEIL OF
STERILITY

The case of the unhinged knee was a high-visibility cover-up that was hidden from public view by a plaster cast.

Most surgical errors are committed behind operating-room doors where mistakes have few witnesses, where only the members of the surgical team ever know what happened. Meanwhile, the patient lies there, unconscious, having assumed prior to surgery that the doctor will observe the Hippocratic Oath and do his best—and that, indeed, the doctor knows what he is doing. But how can the patient know for sure? With whom should a skeptic check to be sure his doctor is competent? With another doctor? Seldom does an outsider have the opportunity to stand, as I have done, behind the veil of sterility and see what it hides.

Time and again I watched the mutual protection league swing into action, to the extent that I shuddered for the human being lying helpless and unaware on the operating table.

One afternoon late in 1974, Dr. Walter DeYoung—as I call him—telephoned to say he had a patient, a man in his seventies, with an infected total hip. "I'm going to take out the prosthesis," he said. "Meet me in the OR on Tuesday at one o'clock." I wondered why he had scheduled a hip case for such a late hour.

That procedure is usually scheduled first thing in the morning when the operating room is newly scrubbed and disinfected, and least likely to transmit infection-bearing organisms from other cases into the patient's open incision.

As if to read my mind, he explained: "The OR is very quiet after lunch, and I want to do this procedure when the heavy traffic is over."

Several days later I arrived at the appointed hour, and made my usual detour by way of the administration office—to let them know I was in the building. The hospital administrator insisted that salesmen check in with him or his assistant; mainly, I think, because both men disliked salesmen and wanted to keep some control over their activities. Next I walked past the directress of nursing's office on the second floor, and on to the operating room. As DeYoung and I were putting on greens, I noticed that no other surgeon was present.

"Who's assisting on the case?" I asked.

"You are."

The impact of what was happening suddenly hit: DeYoung wanted as few witnesses as possible to the fact that he was operating on an infected total hip. The only bystanders were the operating-room supervisor, the scrub nurse, the anesthesiologist, and me. This was a direct violation of hospital practice that whenever a patient is given general anesthesia an assistant surgeon would be present.

The first time I saw the patient, he was on the operating table, sedated and unaware of the drama unfolding across the room, where the anesthesiologist and DeYoung were deep in discussion about how to anesthetize him.

"This guy has a pacemaker. What are we going to do?" the anesthesiologist asked DeYoung.

"We can't put him out. We'll have to give him a local," DeYoung said, referring to a spinal block which numbs all feeling below the waist.

I thought the conversation odd. The method of anesthesia in a major—and even a minor—surgical procedure is usually determined well ahead of time. This is especially true when there are potential complications. The pacemaker meant this patient had heart-rhythm disturbances and other problems that might have triggered an adverse or even fatal reaction to a general anesthetic. He could have gone into arrythmia, in which the heart beats irregularly. He could have gone into cardiac arrest, in which the heart stops beating altogether. Had these disasters occurred, I would have been of no help whatsoever because my knowledge of the cardiovascular system is nil. I felt that he should have had a cardiologist assisting in this case. I also suspected why no cardiologist was present: nobody had bothered to look at the patient's chart beforehand to see that he had a pacemaker.

The anesthesiologist prepared to inject the patient in the back to give the local anesthetic. He was so thin and emaciated from an insufficient diet, and the anesthesiologist was so inept, that he had to poke the patient four times with the needle. All the while he murmured, trying to tell the anesthesiologist that it hurt. And as I watched this terrible scene, the thought that kept running through my mind was: "God forbid the man dies on the operating table."

During the operation, the patient fell into a light slumber. I am sure he had no recall later of what transpired. Dr. DeYoung opened the old incision, which had not healed well and was inflamed to a bright pink along the scar. I had never seen an infected hip before, and as the skin and muscle layers parted under DeYoung's knife, I felt sick. I saw not the healthy pinks and reds of tissue and blood, but a thick milky-white residue of pus inside the hip cavity, proving that DeYoung's diagnosis of an infected hip was absolutely correct. After cutting the wire that held the greater trochanter, DeYoung took an osteotome and pried the head of the femoral prosthesis out of the plastic cup. At DeYoung's request, I tapped the femoral prosthesis out with a mallet.

"How should we remove the cup?" DeYoung asked.

"I think if we tap around the rim with an osteotome, it should come out easily," I replied.

When the cup popped out, with cement attached in one piece, pus oozed from the acetabulum. We cleaned up the cavity with large spoonlike curettes as best we could and put the pus in a specimen bottle for analysis in the pathology lab. Then DeYoung and I, our four hands working in unison, started chipping cement from the femoral canal. We trimmed the rough edges on top of the femur, and DeYoung did what is known as a Girdlestone procedure or "hanging hip." This procedure, in essence, leaves the patient walking on his or her muscles. No bone remains to connect hip and leg, and the latter swings in a kind of limbo, with only the ligaments and muscles holding the joint together. Yet patients somehow manage to do well in this condition. One leg is shorter than the other, but the procedure relieves pain, and the patient can walk with the aid of a cane or crutch. Sometimes the lesser trochanter, which protrudes on the inner side of the femur, rides up against the base of the pelvis and helps brace the leg. The Girdlestone procedure, named after a doctor who used it fifty years ago to treat tuberculosis of the hip, is essentially a salvage operation when other treatments have failed.

The infected hip case took about one and a half hours. As we emerged from the operating room, the hallways contained one-third the bustle of the early morning. No doctors were around; most were holding office hours or playing golf. When I reached the locker room, the beeper I had left with my street clothes was signaling me to call my office. My secretary told me to make an emergency delivery of Steinmann pins to a hospital in Port Jefferson, Long Island. I borrowed a box of pins from the operating-room supervisor, grabbed my clothes from the locker, threw them over my arm, and ran downstairs to my car, still wearing blood-soaked greens and shoe covers. While I stopped for a traffic light, I pulled on my sports jacket over my greens.

When I arrived at the hospital the operating-room supervisor said, "Where have you been?"

"Would you believe I've been working in my garden?"

"Not unless you have people buried in your garden."

"Here are your Steinmann pins. I'm going to play golf."

Whereupon I drove over to the Harbor Hills Country Club, also in Port Jefferson, changed clothes, and played eighteen holes of golf. As I putted around the course, I pondered the reasons for the hush-hush surgery. One was obvious: no surgeon wants word of an infected hip to get around. It could kill the patient, or cause the leg to be amputated. It could lead to a malpractice suit. It could lead to loss of staff privileges, which means the surgeon could no longer practice medicine in that hospital.

There was another reason for the surgery-in-secret, and DeYoung and I talked about it earlier that day. He was afraid that another surgeon, a professional rival, might try to make a major issue of the case and convince the hospital administration that only he should be allowed to do total hip surgery in the hospital, thereby depriving DeYoung of a significant source of income. In that area of Long Island the orthopedic surgeons all vied for the same patients. Given the competition, I could understand why DeYoung elected to operate in secrecy, even though I did not approve.

Yet I felt that an infected hip of itself was no indictment of DeYoung. Infections caused by staphylococcal and other bacterial contaminants are among the foremost dangers of total hip surgery, and often develop as many as eight years later. The hip procedure is lengthy, the incision large. Many complex instruments rout about inside the body. Infection also depends upon the patient's general physical condition. But to conceal infection to the point of not bringing in an assistant surgeon qualified to handle the patient's heart condition to me was wrong.

Another facet of the cover-up was far more serious than wheeling a patient into surgery at 1 P.M., when nobody else was around. The patient's first hip prosthesis had been installed at another hospital earlier that year. Had he been admitted to that same hospital, the reason for the latest surgery—infection resulting from the first procedure—would have shown clearly in the hospital records. By admitting him to another hospital, there would be no cross-reporting, and the fact that a postoperative infection had occurred would go unnoticed.

Hospitals take such elaborate precautions to prevent post-op infections that the uninitiated might well wonder how they could possibly occur, especially in total hip surgery. Here is how the nurses at one hospital prepared an operating room for this procedure. The day before the case, the nurses close the operating room around 2 P.M. at the latest, then transfer other cases so that the room remains unused until the hip operation. Under optimum conditions, all the equipment needed is already in the room and no additional items are brought in once the operation starts. The nurses assigned to the case wipe the instrument stands, stools, tables, anesthesia machine, operating table, lights, shelves, special machinery, and instruments with large gauze pads soaked with alcohol. The instruments for the procedure are assembled and sterilized the night before and left in an instrument room adjoining the OR. When the room is ready, it is sealed off with tape placed diagonally across the door. Nobody is permitted to enter until the next morning, when the nurses return at about seven o'clock and rewipe all the items in the room about an hour before surgery. Again, they seal the operating-room door with a piece of tape marked DO NOT ENTER. To discourage spectators, they cover the window in the operating-room door with a towel. The night before a total hip case, the nurses also set the thermostat to about 65 degrees so that the methylmethacrylate cement will not set too fast in the warm air. The tape remains on the door until the patient and the instruments are brought in. The doctor then scrubs his hands, prepares the patient's hip area, returns to the sinks, scrubs his hands and arms for another five to ten minutes, returns, and puts on a sterile surgical gown and double gloves (in case one rips). His nose is already covered with one or two masks to eliminate that source of germs.

Meanwhile, elaborate steps are taken to protect the patient against infection. The night before surgery he showers with Phisohex, an antiseptic soap. Several hours before surgery, he usually receives antibiotics by mouth. A nurse shaves the hip area before surgery from waist to knee. To keep any cuts or scratches from providing a medium for bacteria to grow, she scrubs the entire hip area with an antiseptic, Betadine. The incision area is then cleaned with alcohol, dried, covered with plastic Vidrape, and covered with sterile sheets so that only the operative site remains in sight. Once the hip is opened, the wound is flushed periodically with an antiseptic solution.

Infection is a microscopic matter, with bacteria-laden dust particles, carried by air currents into the incision, a prime source of contamination. A surgeon's hand movements or conversation increase the dust count in the room. The opening and closing of the operating-room door creates a veritable dust storm of bacteria. Hair and skin particles dropping from the bodies of the operating team also cause contamination.

Dr. John Charnley's solution to the vexing infection problem is to banish extraneous people from the OR, encase surgeons in plastic, make them breathe through hoses leading out of the room, and surround the entire surgical team by a twenty-by-twenty-foot sealed enclosure fed with filtered air.

What I often witnessed, however, fell far short of Charnley's ideal. In the operating room described above, there are three doors leading to the scrub sinks, the autoclave area, and the main corridor. The latter usually remained shut throughout an entire case. Yet I have seen the door between the scrub sink and the operating room constantly swing open and shut, and even stand open during a procedure.

I have seen circulating nurses amble in and out. I have seen other doctors wander in to chat with the surgeons—who are ultimately responsible for maintaining sterility—about a forthcoming conference, the price of homes, or some other trivial subject.

I have seen the anesthesiologist—who is responsible not only for putting the patient to sleep but also for making sure he wakes up again—leave the room for coffee or a cigarette. A circulating nurse would retrieve him because the surgeon needed him to monitor the patient's blood pressure when the cement was placed into the acetabulum or medullary canal.

I have seen, halfway through a procedure, the anesthesiologist sit back with his mask resting on his top lip because it irritated the bridge of his nose.

I have seen one scrub nurse relieve another in the middle of an operation so the first could take a lunch break.

Despite the best efforts of the hospital staff to create an uncontaminated environment for the patient, members of the surgical team are frequently not only careless but neglectful of sterile procedure. Nobody complains or tries to enforce the rules because any offender is offset by another person who has violated sterile procedure, who, in turn, is covered by a third person who has done the same. And it is difficult not to be drawn into the web of violations.

A case in point: An orthopedic surgeon once invited me to watch him replace an old Street elbow prosthesis with a new-type total elbow. The night before the operation, the surgeon—Matthew Pilsudski, I will call him—invited me to his house. I brought an elbow complete with implant that I had prepared in my garage, but he had other things in mind.

"Bill," he said, "I want you to do me a favor."

"What do you want, Doctor?"

"I am the first surgeon in this area who is doing one of these total elbows, right?"

"Yes, sir, you're the first."

"Well, I have a Nikon camera, and I would like you to scrub in, and after we're into the case, I want you to break scrub and take some pictures." He wanted photographs of the entire procedure to illustrate a paper he planned to write for a medical magazine.

"Do you know how to operate a Nikon?" he asked.

"No, I don't." So he spent the next hour teaching me how to operate the camera. As I was leaving, he made another request: "I don't want the others to know I want the pictures. Bring the camera in and say you're taking pictures for your company's public relations, okay?"

The next morning I arrived at the hospital about fifteen minutes before the case, which was scheduled for eight o'clock. Dr. Pilsudski—who to my knowledge had never been on time for a case—arrived on time for a change. First thing he asked was, "Do you have the camera?"

"Yes."

"Good. Ask the OR supervisor for permission to take pictures."

I went to her office and told her my company wanted to photograph the procedure because it was a new type of prosthesis. She agreed, even though the camera was an unsterile object that could not go into the autoclave. The assistant surgeon had arrived and as we stood at the scrub sinks, another minor drama in surgical procedure began to unfold.

While we brushed our knuckles and arms, I suddenly noticed the OR supervisor come up behind Dr. Pilsudski and pretend to bump into him accidentally. She held a swab in her hand because she was trying to culture Dr. Pilsudski without his knowing it. He had large boils all over his neck that she had apparently suspected for months might harbor staph infection. It was hospital practice to periodically culture the operating-room staff, but the unwritten law of the primacy of the surgeon did not permit an operating-room supervisor to demand a staph culture from him. So she used another tactic.

"Oh, excuse me, Doctor," she said, and quietly dropped the swab in her pocket. She gave me a keep-your-mouth-shut look, which I was delighted to honor because I knew she was trying to take good care of her operating room.

The total elbow case—Dr. Pilsudski's first—was not one of his best operations. The old prosthesis remained stuck in the patient's arm, and after considerable tapping with a surgical mallet, Dr. Pilsudski managed to remove it, along with a small piece of the humerus or upper arm bone. He asked what he should do.

"Just file down the bone," I suggested, "and when the new prosthesis goes in, it won't matter."

Dr. Pilsudski's real concern, however, was not the elbow but the Nikon:

"Get a shot from over here, Bill."

"Get this angle."

"Get a picture of us doing" this—or that.

I estimate that we spent thirty additional minutes of operative time just setting up different shots, posing the patient's arm and their hands next to it. My main role was taking a roll of 35-millimeter color photographs, although later in the procedure I scrubbed and helped hold the prosthesis while the cement set. At that point the circulating nurse became the photographer.

After the case, Dr. Pilsudski asked me to have the photos developed and bring him copies. I had them processed, but never gave him copies. He apparently forgot about them because I photographed him in other, more successful, cases after that. Several weeks later the OR supervisor told me that the culture of Dr. Pilsudski's neck had miraculously disappeared from the pathology lab. Thus, she never learned whether Dr. Pilsudski harbored staph infection, and she never found another way to culture his neck surrepetitiously.

Another, more unusual case of surgical contamination took place in late September 1974. About a week before the case the operating-room supervisor, whom I will call Sarah Burke, called and ordered some Kuntscher intramedullary nails, which are long spikes the surgeon inserts into the femoral canal to hold a fracture together. But nails were not all that Sarah wanted. She called to tell me that Tom Merriman and Myron Eckhardt (not their real names) were scrubbing on this case together. "You know how they hate each other's guts," she reminded me, and asked if I could attend the operation and act as a buffer between them, "to keep them both calmed down." The feud was an ancient one.

Having accepted the role of intermediary, I decided I had better learn more about the case. Dr. Eckhardt told me that the patient was a young man whose femur had been fractured in an automobile accident. He had been admitted to the emergency room, where Dr. Merriman treated him and later recommended surgery. The boy's parents, however, wanted a second opinion, and consulted Dr. Eckhardt, who also recommended surgery to treat the fracture. The parents by then felt obligated to have both surgeons present, little realizing the situation they were creating. With two surgeons on the case, the next question was: who would be in charge, and who would assist? The family chose Eckhardt.

On the morning of the surgery, I arrived in the operating room at about seven-thirty. I was standing in the hallway when Dr. Eckhardt arrived. Next Merriman arrived, and the three of us scrubbed, put on gowns and gloves, and began the case. I immediately noticed that Dr. Merriman had decided to keep a very low profile and let Eckhardt preside. The reason for this, I have always suspected, is that Dr. Eckhardt, in a display of surgical one-upmanship, chose a Kuntscher nail because he was familiar with implanting it and knew that Dr. Merriman was not. This gave Eckhardt a psychological advantage over Merriman.

Eckhardt made a five-inch incision in the side of the patient's leg, parallel to the femur, starting just below the hip. Merriman and I held retractors as Eckhardt began working on the leg. He attached a medullary reamer to a Hall II air driver, drilled a pilot hole through the top of the femoral neck near the greater trochanter, and reamed down the medullary canal to make room for the Kuntscher nail that would hold the fracture together. The X rays had indicated what size nail he needed, but when he tapped it several inches into the canal, it was too tight against the wall of the femur. After some coaxing with an extractor, he managed to remove the nail. Eckhardt seemed aggravated that the first nail was the wrong size, because these devices are far harder to remove than to insert.

At this point another source of aggravation appeared: Eckhardt needed an instrument that should have been on the scrub nurse's table but was not. This instrument, a periosteal elevator, is used to scrape fibrous tissue that grows on the outside of a bone. A few minutes later the circulating nurse brought in a new set of orthopedic instruments containing the periosteal elevator, and Eckhardt resumed scraping the bone.

Suddenly, she came running back into the room.

"Stop everything," she said. "Those instruments are not sterile!"

"What do you mean, not sterile?" Eckhardt said.

"We thought the autoclave was on, but it wasn't. Somebody forgot to turn it on. Stop what you're doing and don't touch a thing."

Eckhardt very carefully set down the periosteal elevator he had been using, and the circulating nurse took off his gloves and removed the instruments from the table. Merriman and I also stood motionless with our hands in the air while the circulating nurse stripped off our gowns and gloves. The three of us waited helplessly while she returned the instruments to the autoclave to sterilize them. Meanwhile, she changed our gloves and pinned sterile towels on our gowns with clamps, to cover the areas where the instruments might have touched. She rolled a sterile stockinette up Eckhardt's right arm and fastened it at his shoulders with a towel clamp. About five minutes later, the circulating nurse returned with the instruments. They were red-hot, and the scrub nurse had to dip them in sterile saline to try to cool them.

Now entered the main villain of the case: a common housefly. It buzzed around the room and finally landed on the sterilized gown I had just put on. Then it hopped over to Dr. Eckhardt's gown, contaminating it as well. We all watched with a growing sense of horror as it landed on Dr. Merriman's head and then dropped down to the bridge of his glasses. Dr. Eckhardt, who had marshaled his resources, picked up a can of aerosol spray that is used to stick plastic Vidrapes on the patient's skin and sprayed Merriman square in the face.

"What the fuck did you do that for?" Merriman cried.

Eckhardt—who I am sure meant no malice, despite the rancor between the two men—replied, "I was just trying to catch the fly." Eckhardt missed the fly, but not Merriman's glasses, which were completely fogged up. The circulating nurse came to his aid and wiped them off on her skirt. The fly continued its odyssey around the room, contaminating everything it touched, including the patient's open wound. I assume it wanted a taste of blood before visiting another operating room, where it went upon leaving ours.

For the third time we changed gowns, gloves, and masks, and resumed work on the patient. So far, sterility and other mishaps had delayed the case at least an hour.

Meanwhile, the relationship between Eckhardt and Merriman had not warmed after Eckhardt shot Merriman in the glasses. In fact, most of Eckhardt's comments were directed at me. "Bill, hold this for me. Help me get the nail down here." Eckhardt asked me to place my hands inside the patient and hold the two fragmented ends of the femur with a Lowman bone clamp while he drove the intramedullary nail into the femur. He then asked me to hold the bone plate against the femur while he drilled holes for attaching the plate. In effect, I had replaced Merriman as the assistant surgeon. He stood across the table and occasionally held retractors.

We finished the procedure without having a major confrontation between the two men. In fact, the two doctors acted like gentlemen despite the incident with the aerosol. As Merriman and I were walking down the hall afterward, he said, "What a stupid putz! How the hell could he shoot me in the eyes with that stuff! Thank God we're out of there. I'll never scrub with that guy again."

I never learned whether the patient suffered harm from flyspecks in his open leg wound. Had a postoperative infection developed, I expect that the patient, like the man with the infected hip, might well have been admitted to another hospital rather than the one where the infection took place. If such patients never return, the hospital can report a very low postoperative infection rate for there is no cross-reporting. Thus the staffs at various institutions cannot connect the case with the earlier surgery at another hospital. And because some hospitals have nearly identical medical staffs, it is a simple matter for a surgeon who has privileges at two hospitals to admit a patient to one for the initial procedure and, if complications arise, to send that patient to the second hospital the next time around.

A fly in the operating room is what Lloyd's of London would call an uninsurable "act of God." I am not so sure about the mouse case. I heard about it from a salesman who later worked for me. Once, while observing a total hip case, he was at the side of the operating room talking to another salesman. Suddenly he looked down and spied, just off his left foot, a dead mouse. He nudged it with his toe. Sure enough, it was dead. He then nudged his companion, who looked down in disbelief. They called for the circulating nurse, who picked the mouse up in a towel and carried it from the operating room. The mouse case could be considered a minor violation of sterile procedure, since the creature was outside the immediate operative field. But nobody could be sure where the mouse had been before he died.

Still, the fly case, and perhaps even the mouse case, are examples not of surgical incompetence but of bad luck. No surgeon could have prevented a fly from invading his operating room. And the steps taken afterward to re-establish sterility were prompt and appropriate. Even the unsterilized instruments in that case were the result of forgetfulness. The other incidents, however—the conscious violations like the camera in the operating room, traffic in and out of the room, extra visitors, inattentive nurses and surgeons, the masks drooping under doctor's noses, uncultured sores on a surgeon's neck—these, I think, show a significant gap between the rules and reality of sterile procedure. Even worse, the surgery conducted in secrecy to hide a postoperative infection probably resulted from such carelessness. Worst of all is the concealment of such instances by transferring patients with postoperative infections to a different hospital when further treatment is needed. All this and more is hidden by the veil of sterility.

NINE
THE
MIRANDO CASE

The case that brought my name before the public began on May 21, 1975, when Franklin Mirando, then a forty-two-year-old gasoline service station owner from Nesconset, Long Island, tripped over a hose. Like all the other names used in this chapter, Mirando's name is real. At first, he felt pain in his knee. Bathing it in hot tubs did not provide relief; the pain spread and grew worse. Finally he went to Smithtown General Hospital, where he was treated by the chief of orthopedic surgery, Dr. David Lipton, who later told him that his injury had triggered arthritis of the hip and that only an artificial one could relieve his pain. Mirando consented. The operation was scheduled for July 3, 1975, at Smithtown General Hospital.

Several days before the surgery, Dr. Lipton's secretary called my wife at home and left word that Dr. Lipton wanted to see me before the operation. When I went to his office he told me that in ordinary circumstances, the patient was too young for a total hip implant. But it was the only way he could continue to manage his gas station.

On the morning of the case, I arrived at Smithtown General around seven-thirty and greeted the operating-room supervisor,

Lorna Salzarullo. Soon after we put on scrub clothes, Dr. Lipton joined us in the doctor's lounge. At about seven-forty-five, Dr. Harold Massoff, Lipton's partner, arrived.

The next thing I knew, Lipton was asking me to scrub in case he needed assistance. So I went to the scrub sinks. I had not intended to scrub and was planning merely to advise the nurses on the proper use of the Charnley instruments my firm had loaned the hospital for the procedure.

When the case began at 8 A.M., Lipton was standing out in the main corridor. Dr. Massoff made the initial incision in Mirando's right hip and followed the usual Charnley steps: He removed the greater trochanter and femoral head. Through the blood I could see that the bone appeared to be deteriorated and arthritic.

When Lipton joined us in the operating room, he put on gloves and started helping Dr. Massoff, who had reamed the acetabulum and was ready to position the cup. Massoff took the Charnley positioning instrument, moved it around in the cup, and asked me whether it looked all right. "The cup looks too anteverted," I said—it angled too far upward. There was some disagreement. The opinion of the doctors prevailed, and Massoff left the cup in the patient in an anteverted position. Massoff then reamed out the femoral canal, inserted the cement, and positioned the femoral prosthesis. As they did a trial reduction (a test of how the prosthesis worked) I noticed the leg moved in all directions as it should, although the implant itself looked loose and wobbly. They had not accepted my comments about positioning the cup. Besides, it was a sunny July day and I wanted to hit some golf balls at the Harbor Hills Country Club. Since there was no further service I would perform, I simply announced: "I am leaving."

The golf course is about fifteen minutes away by car. I traveled State Route 25A, an old back road that passes through several eighteenth-century-type villages. Normally, I would have driven slowly and enjoyed the view, because I like old buildings. That day I plowed straight ahead toward the golf course. At the clubhouse restaurant, I remember ordering my usual, a Reuben sandwich, playing solitaire, losing, and hoping some other golfers would show up for a game. Nobody did, and finally I asked the caddy to put my clubs on the golf cart. Out on the first hole, relaxed at last, surrounded by green grass and sunlight, I decided to forget about the morning's surgery.

The second hole is a par three, and I recall hitting the ball into a sand trap, wedging it out, and sinking a four-foot putt to make par. I was feeling good as I hit a long drive off the third tee. Suddenly I noticed a cart moving toward me. It was a member of the club staff and he told me: "Bill, there is an urgent message for you from Smithtown General Hospital. They want to speak to you immediately."

I jumped into my cart and rode back to the clubhouse, where I called my office. "What's the problem?" I asked my secretary, Shirley.

"A patient has dislocated in the recovery room at Smithtown General."

I called the operating-room secretary at Smithtown. "We're waiting for you. Can you get over here right away?" she asked.

I ran to my car, still wearing golf clothes, and drove back to the hospital. As I parked outside the emergency room, a guard objected: "You can't park here."

"There's an emergency in the operating room, and I'm leaving the car here, so tough."

Upstairs, the operating-room secretary told me, "Hurry up, get into greens!" As I exited from the doctor's lounge into the main corridor, Lorna Salzarullo, the operating-room supervisor, was walking down the hall toward me: "Thank God you're here!"

It was about 1:30 P.M. when I walked into the operating room and saw Lipton and Massoff standing there. The two surgeons held their arms up in the air, waiting for the scrub nurse to put gloves on them. "Go scrub," Lipton said. "Hurry up, we've got a problem here." While I was at the sinks, he kept looking in and saying, "Come on, hurry, get in here." I could still see into the operating room through a door with a glass window. Massoff was clipping open the stitches he had made less than three hours earlier. When I returned to the OR, the hip was open. Round 2 of the historic Mirando case had begun.

Massoff, from his post at the patient's right hip, told Lipton: "Maybe we ought to give this guy a hanging hip." Lipton, who was at Massoff's right, said, "No, he came in here for a new hip. Let's send him home with one." I stood between the two surgeons. Meanwhile, Brian O'Hare, a new salesman of mine in training, was standing at the side of the room, outside the sterile area, watching the operation at a distance.

Massoff cut the wires holding the greater trochanter and pulled them out. When he tried to remove the femoral prosthesis—tap, tap, tap—it would not budge. He asked me to remove it. I took a mallet, and, after several tries, the prosthesis came out. Then Lipton, who had been watching Massoff, made a decision: "Harold, go back and do office hours. Bill and I will finish the case."

Thus Dr. Harold Massoff left the operating room.

Lipton moved into his place, and I moved into Lipton's.

The marathon began with Lipton removing cement from the femoral canal. He sat on his stool, chipping away with an osteotome. Suddenly, from my lower left, I heard him curse to himself.

"What's the matter?" I asked.

"The whole thing has fallen apart!"

I looked into the hip cavity and saw that Lipton had shattered the upper end of the femur into several splits on the inner side.

He rose from his stool and said, "What are we going to do now?"

"Dave," I said, "we can take out the cement and reapproximate the bone. We can wrap Parham bands around the femur or we can use eighteen-gauge surgical wire."

"You do it," he ordered. And so I sat on his round, stainless-steel stool, still warm from his body, and he stood behind me and watched. I looked at the scrub nurse and said, "Give me a pair of rongeurs." I took the plierlike instrument and, with its sharp pointed ends, picked loose cement fragments from the femoral shaft.

No instructions that I knew of had ever been written for the removal of hardened bone cement in this type of situation. I would have to play it by ear. I asked the circulating nurse to bring me some medullary reamers and an orthotome air drill with a nine-sixteenth-inch bit. But because the femoral shaft was already damaged, I could not use the drill and reamers except to attack the most stubborn pieces of cement. The hand tools—the osteotome and rongeurs—would be slower, but safer. It was going to be a tedious, step-by-step process of wedging the osteotome between the cement and femoral shaft, thereby creating a gap to get the fragments out. The fact that the femoral shaft was shattered did make access somewhat easier because of the wider entrance. One piece of cement, however, was lodged far down the shaft, beyond the reach of my tools.

I lengthened the incision by two inches and asked the scrub

nurse for the air drill. With it I drilled four holes in the femur as the markers for a window I intended to cut with a small osteotome. I connected the holes and fashioned a small squarish opening in the femur so I could insert a punch and push the cement up from below. I dropped the piece of femur into a specimen dish so I could replace it later on. Lipton stood behind my right shoulder and asked from time to time, "How're we doing, Bill?" "That looks good." "Good, Bill." Later he moved around to the left side of the operating table to help me retract tissue.

The process seemed endless, and bleeding continued to hamper visibility. Far worse, it threatened the life of the patient who, by then, had received numerous transfusions. Too much blood might have made him "wash out." He had been under anesthesia from 8:15 A.M. until around noon that morning. Now, in Round 2, he had been under at least since one-thirty, when I returned from the golf course. It was then nearly four o'clock. When a person is asleep that long, he sometimes never wakes up.

At long last, the cement was out. The job had taken one and a half hours. The next problem was putting the upper end of the femur back together. I asked for some Parham bands—flat stainless-steel bands about an eighth of an inch wide by six inches long with a slot in one end through which the band threads and holds against itself. First I placed the new prosthesis in the shaft to be sure no cement remained. Then I restructured the femur, making sure the splits in the bone, which measured from half an inch to an inch and a half, fit together like a jigsaw puzzle. The job was nervewracking: I feared the bone might break apart at any moment. I encircled it with several Parham bands, drawing them as tight as possible so the fragments would hold together. Then I took a rasp and very carefully smoothed the inside of the femur.

Now that the fracture was stabilized, I turned to Lipton and said, "As long as we're doing this, why don't we do the whole damn thing over and take out the cup." As I had suspected that morning, it was too anteverted. I pried the acetabular cup loose with an osteotome, and it popped out. Meanwhile, Lipton mixed some new cement. When it no longer stuck to his gloves, the sign that it was ready, I shaped it like a flat hamburger patty and pressed it into the acetabulum. I positioned the new cup, and Lipton curetted the excess cement from around the edges. He mixed another batch of cement. I packed it into the femoral canal and very carefully inserted the new femoral prosthesis while holding the upper end of the femur with my left hand. Then Lipton and I built up the missing top of the femur with cement to give the prosthesis a platform to ride on.

At this point Lipton and I traded places. He reclaimed his stool and rewired the greater trochanter back to the femur. I assisted by twisting the wires into a knot and bending them back into the bone. When we put the leg through a complete range of motion, the new joint was perfect. Not merely good, but perfect. After placing a Hemovac drain in the wound, Lipton sewed it up while I tied and cut knots. Lipton bandaged the patient and placed an abduction pillow between his legs to keep him from moving around and accidentally dislocating the hip.

It was nearly 8 P.M. when we left the operating room, Lipton to see the patient's family, I to see mine. For nearly twelve hours, Franklin Mirando had been in surgery, including the interlude in the recovery room. But at least he had been unconscious.

For me the experience had been a battle. The muscles in my back were so knotted from the long hours on the stool that it was agony when I walked. I looked at my greens. They were red and soaked with blood. It was all over my chest, on my thighs, lower legs, feet. The blood had soaked through my shoe covers and onto my loafers. Then I heard a squish and realized that I even had blood inside my shoes.

Heading home in my car, feeling totally wrung out, I suddenly had an urge to return to the Harbor Hills Country Club. After what had happened that day, I had to wind down before going home. As I sat in the lounge, I said to myself, "You know, Bill, you have just finished one of the nicest pieces of surgery you have ever seen or done."

It was one of the greatest experiences of my life. But I had no idea as to what the repercussions of this experience would be.

TEN

THE ORTHOPEDIC GAME

The Mirando case had an unhappy outcome. It should not have surprised me.

Ordinarily my contact with a patient began the moment I entered the operating room and ended when I walked out. I seldom knew the patient's name, and did not learn Mirando's until long afterward. Still, I usually knew how a case turned out because in orthopedic surgery the postoperative X rays show—as they do not in many other branches of medicine—what the surgeon has accomplished. If the X rays reveal that the femoral prosthesis sits securely in the cup, or that the two parts of an artificial knee fit together and align correctly with the bone, the surgery most likely has been a success.

Because Franklin Mirando's case had special personal significance, I asked at least three times how the patient was doing. "Fine, fine," was the reply. "He's doing just great." Not until October 1977, more than two years after the surgery, did I learn to my great distress that Mr. Mirando was *not* doing fine. In fact, he claimed he was in great pain, and was confined most of the time to a wheelchair. His right leg, he said, was two inches shorter than his left, and he filed a forty-million-dollar malpractice claim against Drs. Lipton and Massoff. During the ensuing controversy, my role in putting Mr. Mirando's hip back together was unveiled. For this he has expressed gratitude, and has credited me with keeping the disaster that occurred on July 3, 1975, from turning out even worse. But I am ahead of my story.

When the Mirando case became public knowledge, many people asked, "How could this have happened?" So far I have recounted—from doctoring horses, to selling artificial hips, to implanting them in cadavers, to implanting them in live people—how *I* was able to perform as I did in surgery. But how could others—orthopedic surgeons at the pinnacle of their professions, anesthesiologists, operating-room supervisors, scrub nurses, circulating nurses, hospital administrators, and the rest—how could *they* have permitted such a situation?

The answer begins with hospitals such as Smithtown. Consider the history of this institution. Smithtown General opened its doors in 1961 to serve the thriving middle-class community of Smithtown, Long Island, where average incomes range from $15,000 to $18,000 per year. Smithtown must have been a lovely town back in 1945, before the town fathers succumbed to vendors of aluminum signs, shopping malls, and endless stretches of tract housing. As those "improvements" were made, the wage-earners of this tinsel town crammed the 6 A.M. commuter trains bound for Manhattan. Their migrations attracted the attention of one Dr. Anton Notey, his real name, who reasoned that while the inhabitants of Smithtown might leave to work and play, they would return home whenever they got sick. With an eye on the census, which had reached 46,000 by the late 1950s, he proposed that a local hospital be built in Smithtown. The 274-bed institution, which opened in 1961, was financed fifty-one percent by Dr. Notey, fifteen percent by a group of about forty doctors in the Smithtown area, and the remainder by outside investors, also doctors. Dr. Notey, a general practitioner, was also principal owner of another hospital, three nursing homes (which supplied patients for his hospitals), and a linen service (which washed sheets for his nursing homes and hospitals). I would not have been surprised to learn that he owned a mortuary to complete the eternal chain.

A footnote on Notey: In March 1978 he was accused, in a twenty-four-count indictment, of stealing $1.8 million from Smithtown General, Medicaid, and private insurers. Reporter Neill Rosenfeld of *Newsday* called the amount "the most anyone has been accused of taking from or through a single institution in the state." Also charged in a more than forty-count indictment was the Smithtown hospital administrator, John F. Gans. A Suffolk County grand jury accused the two of sending inflated and bogus bills, accepting illegal kickbacks, and operating a facility to launder same.

The Smithtown community continued to grow to the point that the Episcopal Diocese of Long Island decided to build a 300-bed voluntary hospital. The St. John's Smithtown Hospital opened in December 1966 about one mile from Smithtown General. While the latter is a profit-making institution, owned and operated by doctors, and St. John's is nonprofit, both hospitals exist to sell professional medical services to people who are sick, injured, disabled, and dying.

Yet consider how these two hospitals recruited the doctors who offer those services. Back in the early 1960s, Smithtown General required no more than a license to practice medicine, a curriculum vitae, and letters of reference. The latter usually went unchecked unless the credentials committee had doubts about the applicant.

When St. John's opened in late 1966, some 200 applications flooded in, mostly from physicians who already had privileges to practice at Smithtown. This became the basis for acceptance at St. John's. The mass hiring produced almost virtually identical staffs at the two hospitals. It also brought in some fascinating physicians to the shared staffs of Smithtown General and St. John's. I speak of Dr. Edward Altchek and Dr. Moses Ashkenazy, for example, who arrived in the mid-1960s and who performed the first craniotomy case I ever observed, the one where the saw blade got stuck in the patient's skull. By early 1977 the exploits of these two doctors had become familiar newspaper reading.

Dr. Altchek, a neurosurgeon on the Smithtown and St. John's staffs, admitted in 1976 to having sexually molested at least seven female patients during the preceding three years. After numerous complaints about Altchek's behavior, St. John's finally took disciplinary steps. The hospital allowed him to see patients only when a nurse was escorting him. He was required to report to the lobby of the hospital, announce his presence, and wait for either a nursing supervisor or a floor nurse to come down. Finally, St. John's suspended him from the staff, although he continued to practice at Smithtown and Brookhaven hospitals. Meanwhile, the State of New York investigated his behavior and, in November 1976, decided to revoke his medical license for three years. Yet, less than three weeks before New York revoked it, the State of Michigan granted him a license to practice medicine on the recommendation of three colleagues.

Dr. Moses Ashkenazy's troubles stemmed from allegations that he performed unnecessary and excessive surgery, particularly on patients with sore necks. Eventually two dozen patients sued him for malpractice. They claimed damages ranging from unnecessary surgery to constant pain, partial paralysis, and permanent disablement. One case was settled out of court for $285,000, among the largest awards ever approved in Suffolk County. Dr. David Lipton was a co-defendant in this case, and neither he nor Dr. Ashkenazy would admit to having done the surgery. Dr. Ashkenazy left Smithtown in 1974 and moved to California, with some $28 million in malpractice claims pending against him and a million dollars on prior claims paid out.

Despite the number of malpractice cases against Dr. Ashkenazy, neither Smithtown nor St. John's ever took disciplinary action against him. And no official hospital committee or board ever censured his behavior. At Smithtown, Ashkenazy once had to defend his professional conduct before a large gathering of his colleagues, but this was the extent of peer review of his activities.

Fancier definitions probably exist, but to me the term *peer review* means that a person must be accountable for his actions. At Smithtown and St. John's, whatever kind of review procedures might have existed on paper was, in my opinion, no effective self-policing of medical misconduct. Also, the pressures to keep beds full were so intense that any surgeon who performed frequent surgery helped that hospital survive economically. A doctor who admitted large numbers of patients to Smithtown General or St. John's was not apt to be disciplined or dismissed. For example, Dr. Ashkenazy, who kept many beds full at Smithtown General and St. John's, once left the emergency room unattended and was suspended for a week. Another doctor, who did not hospitalize his patients very often, committed a similar violation and had his privileges revoked.

Among surgeons at other hospitals that I visited, the pressures to fill hospital beds produced intense rivalries. Surgeons watched jealously to see how many total hips, knees, and other prostheses their colleagues ordered from me and from other salesmen. They frequently asked, "How is Dr. Smith doing?" The query was not about Dr. Smith's health but about the number of patients I counted in his waiting room during sales rounds, or the number of total hips he purchased the preceding month.

At extremes the rivalry led to undercutting other doctors, including one's own partners, and to verbal assault in conference and operating rooms. Doctors constantly asked me: "How was that knee case with Dr. X? I hear it didn't go so well." They hoped that I would supply some prurient details, but I invariably pleaded ignorance. I have heard doctors question a colleague's professional competence in orthopedic conferences to the point where two surgeons were literally ready to punch one another in the nose.

Frequently I saw doctors locked in an eternal struggle to be on the emergency-room roster. This was a favorite device for building their practices, since any doctor on call in the hospital emergency room would likely gain that person as a patient. Emergency-room time was a privilege, and some hospitals did not accord it to new physicians. But once on the roster, doctors would virtually lie, cheat, and ingratiate themselves with the emergency-room nurses in order to increase their share of emergency-room time. One orthopedic surgeon, who considered himself quite the ladies' man, courted the nurses until they started recommending him instead of the doctor on call to attend to a case. Finally, other surgeons openly chastised him at orthopedic conferences and tried to have his privileges revoked.

Orthopedic surgeons once banded together to prevent general surgeons from doing orthopedic procedures during emergency-room calls. "We don't do appendectomies or hernias," the orthopods stormed, "so why the hell should you pin a hip?" The orthopods finally convinced the hospital administration to limit general surgeons to caring for fractures, although they wanted that privilege revoked too.

Hospital privileges are another cause of rivalry. They directly affect the amount of money a doctor earns. Every staff physician has a card which states what he is allowed to do in that hospital. Ideally, though not necessarily, this coincides with what he was trained to do. But a doctor who wines and dines the Chief of Surgery and other key people might find that his card lists more privileges than the physician who stays home reading medical journals. So the former's card might say he is qualified to do total hips even though he watched only one as a resident. Working in reverse, the privilege card of another doctor might show that he can perform gall-bladder, hernia, or hemorrhoid procedures, but for anything more complex he must have another surgeon supervising.

Orthopedic surgeons endlessly curry the favors of general practitioners, who are a major source of referral as the first physician the patient usually sees. No fee-splitting occurs, because that practice is illegal. But the parties, dinner invitations, hunting trips, and expensive gifts at Christmastime are all legal ways to enrich the GP for sending the orthopedist his patients.

Many doctors compete for wealthy patients while turning away the poor. I once saw a surgeon at a well-heeled hospital in Suffolk County, Long Island, overprepare for surgery to the point of sterilizing the scrub suits. He was trying to impress a socially prominent patient who might refer her wealthy friends if she was pleased (and might sue him for malpractice if she was not). By contrast, I have seen doctors refuse to sell soft goods—slings, braces, and the like—to patients covered by workmen's compensation, which reimburses the doctor only $26, say, for a knee brace that costs him $22. I have seen supply cabinets in doctors' offices with signs saying, "Do not issue soft goods to workmen's compensation patients," even though these patients need a brace or sling. Such doctors generally send these patients to a surgical supply house for their needs or refuse to treat them altogether.

Perhaps the greatest rivalries center around surgery itself. Surgeons constantly try to sell their services to patients, promising that a certain procedure will relieve a painful leg, restore a stiff arm, or enable them to dance at their daughters' weddings. Franklin Mirando reported that Lipton said he would be back to work several weeks after his artificial hip was installed. In my business, that is called selling. Indeed, many doctors I encountered "sold" hip and knee surgery even though they totally lacked experience to perform it. They sold elbow and ankle procedures even though these devices are highly experimental, with high rates of failure. But these doctors were selling surgery, and there was virtually nothing they would not undertake, especially if they had me standing by. Thus a salesman became a surgeon, but only because the surgeon had become a salesman.

Soft goods—casts, slings, braces, collars, and the like—offered doctors some of the greatest opportunities for sales and profit. As a rule, doctors marked up the soft goods I sold them 250 percent. One of the most popular items is the simple knee brace. For years, doctors would tell a patient with a sprained knee to apply ice packs, elevate the knee, and wrap an elastic Ace bandage around it. No more. The modern treatment is a knee brace, a wrapping with six Velcro closures, and two steel stays that hold the leg extended. This apparatus has several advantages: it never binds or cuts off blood circulation as an Ace bandage does. And it is eligible for Medicare reimbursements. Meanwhile, I charged the doctor $12.50 for the brace. The doctor charged the patient about $35, including office visit, making his total return about $80 on a $12.50 investment.

When the knee brace comes off, the doctor wraps the patient's leg in gauze or an elastic bandage. I have known many a doctor who takes the knee brace home to his wife, who washes it. He then sells it to the next patient with a sprained or injured knee. The patient is so happy to be rid of the brace he does not notice or care that the doctor keeps it. And the patient seldom has the foresight to say, "Doctor, I own that brace. Would you please give it back to me?" Arm slings are also washed and resold, but most of the recycling involves knee braces.

Tennis elbow also provides many opportunities for profit. The classic cure for this affliction is rest and the passage of time, but many patients would take painful elbows to doctors on my calling list who would wrap the joint in three-quarter-inch adhesive tape. But few tennis buffs would be impressed by a doctor who stuck a piece of tape on their elbow and charged them $35. So the doctor does a rain dance around the elbow, orders an X ray, and announces, "You have tendinitis of the elbow, my dear. You will have to rest it." He then produces a tennis-elbow band: a red, white, and blue piece of elasticized cotton webbing with Velcro closures. He wraps the band, which I sell for $1.25, around the elbow like a belt. He charges the patient $5 for the band and $35 for the consultation.

Another profitable item in the orthopedist's armamentarium is the cast. It costs the patient from $75 to $350 and the doctor about $3 for the plaster, which comes in rolls long enough to make several short-arm casts, plus the stockinette which goes between the skin and the cast. To earn his fee, the doctor manipulates the arm a little bit, takes an X ray (which probably costs extra) to make sure the arm is aligned properly, puts the stockinette on the arm, soaks the plaster roll in a basin, and wraps it around the arm. In fifteen minutes it gets hard and he tells the patient to go home and keep his arm elevated. The cast dries out overnight, and the next day he goes to school or work, where all his friends write on it. Six weeks later, the cast comes off. The arm has healed, not by the doctor but by Wolff's Law, which declares that even after a bone stops growing, microscopic changes continuously occur in reaction to stress. This process allows a bone to heal naturally while confined in a cast. In other words, Mother Nature does the real work and never charges a cent.

In general, a doctor charges according to the size, importance, and geographic location of his practice. If he lives in an affluent area like Great Neck, Long Island, he might charge $80 for a special postoperative knee brace that I sell for $22. If he practices in Levittown, he might charge $45 for the same item. An arm sling the doctor purchased from me for $3 might cost the patient $5 or $10. A cervical collar with metal bracing, which costs the doctor $9, might cost the patient $35 and up. As is the case with most medical services, it is a seller's market. The patient must buy these devices from the doctor or surgical supply store at retail price because these are the only outlets, and because Federal law prohibits their sale without a doctor's prescription.

In big-league surgery, a total hip might cost from $2000 to $5000, depending upon the patient's income. A total knee might cost $2500, an elbow $1500. I know one surgeon who charged $5500 for a scoliosis operation to correct severe curvature of the spine. After the procedure he put the patient in a body cast—and would not remove it until the fee was paid in full. An anesthesiologist's bill might run from $200 to $500, an assistant surgeon's fee from $500 to $750. Me they got for free.

Doctors' fees run high because of the exorbitant rates they must pay—up to $50,000 a year in premiums—for malpractice insurance. Fees also run high because of greed and that, in medicine, is nothing new. The archives of York County, Virginia, show that of 145 medical bills recorded between 1637 and 1700, the average charged 752 pounds of tobacco, slightly less than one man could produce in a year. The latest studies of doctor's incomes show they are rising at a faster rate than the incomes of any other occupational group, and on the average are unjustifiably high. The median income of doctors was $63,000 in 1976. Doctors in the Long Island area did substantially better than this: I estimate that the average orthopedic surgeon during my selling days was topping $250,000 a year.

The numbers add up to money medicine, a state of mind that explains why so many surgeons did not refer patients to more qualified colleagues and undertook procedures they were ill prepared to perform, especially when they had me to bail them out.

ELEVEN

ME DOCTOR

Many of the problems in medicine today exist because patients seldom question their doctors or, if they do, they ask about the wrong things. Orthopedics is ripe for malpractice claims because the patient's condition before and after surgery is visible. And malpractice suits often arise when the patient feels the results did not match his hopes, which may never have been attainable in the first place. A patient may come in with a crushed elbow and no movement in that arm. The surgeon opens him up and sees that there is little he can do. Still he does his best. Because of the surgeon's best efforts, the patient regains perhaps forty percent of his elbow function. But he does not feel satisfied, so he tells his lawyer: "Before my accident I could completely extend my arm. Now I can only bend it this far." After investigation, if the lawyer believes malpractice is involved, he may recommend filing a suit.

One doctor installed a total hip in a seventy-five-year-old woman from a nursing home. He did a fine job, in my opinion, but about six months later the woman decided that she had problems with the hip. She sued the doctor for more than $200,000 because she (or more likely her family) did not think she got perfect results. Another total hip patient sued a surgeon because she developed a decubitus ulcer on her heel during the postoperative period. This stemmed not from surgery but from poor nursing care. Still, the insurance company settled out of court for $35,000. The net result of all this litigation is that surgeons charge blockbuster fees for surgery because they cannot otherwise afford to pay blockbuster premiums for malpractice insurance. Then, as I said earlier, the surgeons must sell more surgery to more patients to cover insurance costs.

Meanwhile, the patient who does not sue for malpractice, and he is in the majority, is content to accept whatever the doctor says and does. This unquestioning attitude places doctors on a pedestal and perpetuates something called the MD (Me Doctor) Syndrome, a disease that pervades American medicine. It makes sacred cows of doctors, allows them to enjoy perquisites unknown to the average citizen, and to cover up errors—with the aid of their peers. Worst of all, the MD Syndrome allows doctors to avail themselves of salesmen like me whenever they accept a case they cannot handle.

One favorite Me Doctor technique is to keep medical-equipment salesmen thumbing through last year's magazines two or three hours in the waiting room while the doctor sees patients, makes phone calls, reads X rays, and writes memos. This is understandable, perhaps, when the salesman is on a sales call. But often a doctor asks a salesman to lend him a movie, an assortment of artificial knees, or $5000 worth of instruments for doing a total hip procedure.

A doctor who heard I collected cadaver bones said, "I have a total hip coming up, and I haven't done a Charnley in over a year. I'd like to work on my wiring technique."

"I have femurs and wire and everything you need over at my office," I said.

Several days later he came to my office in my apartment building in Roslyn. He selected a femur from my bone box, and I gave him a saw, power drill, nine-sixty-fourth-inch drill bit, wire, and everything else he would need. I plugged the drill into the only electric outlet in the room, which was near my walnut conference table.

"Are you all squared away?" I asked. "I've got some paperwork in the next room. And, please be careful not to drill a hole in the table."

"Sure, I'll be careful."

From the next room I could hear him drilling, buzzing, and sawing like a busy little beaver. When I returned ten minutes later, five nine-sixty-fourth-inch holes dotted the distal end of my conference table.

The foremost victims of inconsiderate treatment, however, were patients. The Me Doctor Syndrome often makes the doctor lose sight of human values and relegates patients to the role of hips, knees, elbows, shoulders, and ankles, instead of people. I have recounted the times I heard surgeons play rock music in the operating room and nurses chatter about their dinner dates the night before. I have seen anesthesiologists fill out insurance forms while a patient was under anesthesia. I have seen them wander to the corner of the room to converse with a salesman, or leave the room altogether. All this while a human being lies cut open and bleeding on an operating table. Before surgery, I have seen a surgeon walk over to an anesthetized woman lying on an operating table with her body uncovered and put his hand on her breast, fondle it, and say, "Look at the tickets on this one!" And before the case ended, I have seen, time and again, surgeons rush off to conduct office hours, leaving a colleague or a few residents, or in some cases me, to finish the operation.

On the wards, too, callousness was common. I once saw a doctor refuse to make a scoliosis patient more comfortable, even though she lay in a hospital bed asking for help. She was scheduled for surgery in a few days and was encased in a body cast to elongate her curved spine and make it as supple as possible. The patient complained that the cast was irritating the side of her neck. He patted her on the head and said, "Don't worry about it, I'll send an orthopedic technician to cut the cast back for you." In two minutes of his time, he could have done the job with a cast saw.

Again, at Saturday-morning orthopedic conferences at city hospitals and major teaching institutions, I repeatedly saw patients, dressed in surgical gowns that barely covered their bodies, displayed before doctors assembled to discuss their cases. These were "service"—nonpaying—patients, as opposed to private patients. I once saw a teen-age girl brought in after knee surgery. Any girl that age is extremely sensitive about her body. Yet she was covered only by a scanty hospital gown that tied in the back and exposed her to fifteen or twenty gaping men. The fact that they were doctors hardly mattered, for this girl was displayed like a cow on an auction block or, in this case, an examination table.

In a typical conference room, the examination table sits in the middle of the room, surrounded by an X-ray viewbox, a blackboard on wheels, and chairs for the residents and interns. The resident in charge of the patient describes the case and asks for opinions. Then the procession begins. The assembled men of medicine would walk up to her, pinch her knee, and ask her how it felt. Somebody would flip an X ray on the viewer, and she would be escorted to the hallway to await the diagnosis. The attending surgeons would lean toward conservative (nonsurgical) treatments, and the residents toward surgery because they wanted the practice. Finally, the resident in charge would go out and announce the verdict to the patient.

I have seen human beings undergoing this ordeal, frozen with fear, not understanding what the doctors were asking them, not even understanding what was going on. I have seen the question on their agonized faces: "What are they going to do to me?" In women's eyes I have seen tears of embarrassment, in old men's faces tears of pain.

While most hospitals treat private and service patients differently, I know one Chief of Orthopedics who repeatedly reminds his residents, "We have no service patients in this hospital. We have no private patients, either. We just have *patients.*" I only met this man once, but I respect him more than most surgeons, because his statement reflects true concern for the patient.

Dave Lipton, too, is a very compassionate man. I have seen him in the emergency room calming a child with a broken leg, knowing that the child was screaming more in fear than in pain. The true test of compassion is not how a doctor handles children but how he approaches older patients, who tend to be incontinent, hard of hearing, somewhat senile, and resentful that they are no longer self-sufficient. Yet I have seen tremendous displays of empathy for these people—who are the majority of patients in orthopedics. Lipton had a special gift for relating to the aged. He would slow up his pace when talking to them, sound his words carefully, and offer reassurance rather than explanations. I would often see him put his arm around an older patient's shoulder while he spoke.

I know of another doctor who had a patient in the hospital who was slowly suffocating to death from emphysema. Finally, when the man was literally in his last hour of life, the doctor sat with him and cradled him in his arms. As a doctor he could give nothing to the patient. As a human being, he could, and did, give the ultimate gift of caring.

Yet the same doctors who were compassionate in one set of

circumstances could, when infected by the Me Doctor Syndrome, forget the commonality of man and scale the heights of privilege. The medical-equipment industry contributed in major ways toward this situation. Anyone who tried to sell the doctors something gave them, at one time or another, free pens and notepads, free brief cases, free football and theater tickets, and free cocktail parties.

The parking privilege is another familiar privilege; I enjoyed it myself. I had a PHYSICIAN ON CALL sticker on my front windshield which fended off traffic patrolmen writing parking tickets and gained me more than one tankful of gas during the gasoline crisis. One day my friend Wolf asked me to fill up my tank and siphon it into his so he could make sales deliveries. "Wolf, I have a much better idea," I said, and went upstairs and put on my white lab coat and stethoscope. The gas-station attendant was sitting inside his office, with the door closed, when we arrived. He looked as if he never intended to come out. Through the door, I shouted, "I've got an emergency at Eastern Long Island Hospital, and this man needs gas to take me there. Can you help us out?"

"Sure, Doctor, no problem. Just pull up to the pump."

On another occasion I told an attendant at a Texaco station in Glen Cove that I had a kidney transplant to deliver. In my window was an EMERGENCY MEDICAL DELIVERY sticker. The man hesitated, then agreed to fill my tank. By the time he finished, he had four dozen cars lined up at his pump.

I once received a ticket for going 55 mph in a 35-mile zone. I told the state policeman I was en route to a hospital delivering a prosthesis for emergency surgery. He was unmoved and wrote out a ticket anyway. When I arrived, I stopped to see the purchasing supervisor, who took the ticket and said, "Don't worry about it. Just go to court and plead guilty and say you were making an emergency delivery to me. The judge is on the Board of Directors of this hospital." I went to court, and watched the judge mete out $50 fines all morning. When my turn came, I said, "I was making an emergency delivery of a prosthetic device to . . ." Suddenly I could not remember the name of the hospital! The judge said, "—— Hospital, right?"

"Yes, Your Honor."

"I accept your explanation. Case dismissed."

With my borrowed privileges, I parked anyplace I wanted in New York City: in front of fire hydrants, in no-parking zones, in ambulance zones, in emergency entrances, in doctors' parking lots. And why not? I had a PHYSICIAN ON CALL card and—most convincing of all—I was driving a Cadillac!

In most respects, however, I was victim, not beneficiary, of physicians' privilege. For one thing, doctors came to expect freebies up to and including surgical instruments. Given my occupational bias, this is where matters got out of hand. I would sit in a doctor's office with an open case of sample instruments while he examined a pair of Webster needle-holders that cost $50. "You're giving me these, right?" And sometimes, if he was an influential surgeon, I would reply, "Yes." He and his colleagues could have reached into their pockets and handed me enough cash to buy the entire case of instruments. But they would not, because whatever they could get for nothing, they took. A doctor once ordered half a dozen beautiful German-made instruments. He then turned around and sent back several of the instruments, but not through the mail. He expected me to drive back to his office and pick them up, package and mail them back to the manufacturer—with me paying, of course, for the postage. He took six months to pay the $1800 bill for the instruments he kept.

A surgeon who specialized in scoliosis cases extracted the ultimate freebie from me. I was in his office one day showing him a $285 rod bender used to straighten the spine in scoliosis surgery.

"That's some beautiful instrument," he said. "I want that." And he took it right out of my hand.

"Fine," I said. "I'll send you a bill."

"Okay, sure." About two weeks later he received the bill, had the temerity to telephone me and say, "Hey, you *gave* me this instrument!"

"Doctor, you *bought* it, and it costs two hundred eighty-five dollars."

"Bill, I buy all my implants from you. The least you can do is give me the rod bender."

This man earns a six-figure annual income, and he would not pay for a $285 instrument. For three months the manufacturer sent him a bill, which he forwarded to me with a note: "Bill, will you take care of this?" Finally, I ended up paying for the rod bender out of my own pocket.

Other doctors did not filch instruments from me, but merely borrowed them, often returning sets of brand-new instruments looking like they had been overrun by Rommel's tanks. How these doctors managed to inflict such destruction, I do not know. Maybe they bounced the tools around in their car trunks for a day or two, or used them to replace door hinges in their homes, but they certainly did not take care of them.

I wrote earlier about how doctors expected salesmen to convince orthopedic companies to manufacture products they had invented. The electrical cervical collar is a case in point. Here was a device that improved upon the ordinary cervical collar, a brace that immobilizes the head and neck of a patient with whiplash or arthritis, among other conditions. This doctor wanted to wire electric current through the collar to apply heat to the patient's neck as he watched TV or slept at night. The doctor never considered that the patient might spill coffee or beer on the collar and short it out. In fact, he became indignant when I explained that our engineer had told me that it was unsafe.

One company actually manufactured another doctor's brain child: a knee pillow. This device looked like a trapezoidal wedge with a groove at the top. Its sole purpose was to hold the patient's knee up in the air while the surgeon operated on it. The pillow was made of Styrofoam and covered with a special vinyl that would spark under friction and possibly blow the operating room to Kingdom Come. Ordinarily surgeons have an assistant hold the knee, or they place rolled towels under the draping to hold the knee up. This doctor asked the company to pay him a royalty on each pillow sold, and to name the pillow after him. The company declined the latter, and the other condition became moot. Despite the company's best attempts to market it, only one pillow sold in the entire metropolitan New York area, and guess who bought it? Finally, the company sent the doctor a letter saying that because his pillow had not been well received by the orthopedic community, it would be discontinued. The doctor withdrew about $12,000 worth of business from the company.

Withdrawal of business was not uncommon. A doctor in my territory once invented a hinged knee prosthesis that he wanted us to manufacture. I sent the prototype to the home office for evaluation. The same day he called me in and ordered $1800 worth of orthopedic instruments: knee braces, slings, heel protectors, cast boots, all in quantities he was unlikely to use in a year. Then he told me to return every two weeks to keep him in stock. Meanwhile, after examining the knee prosthesis, my company rejected it and sent him a lovely thanks-but-no-thanks letter. Several days later the doctor asked me to stop by his office and reclaim the items he had bought because he no longer needed them. As I went out the door, he announced that he intended to do no more business with us because he considered the company unethical.

The reject list included an artificial patella (kneecap) another doctor wanted my company to make and market for him. If this patella had ever been implanted, the patient would have had a knob on his knee as big as a golf ball and one inch square with rounded edges.

It is generally recognized that the fewer moving parts a prosthesis has, the better it will work. But some doctors do not subscribe to this principle of biomechanics. One surgeon invented a total shoulder with no fewer than _ten_ moving parts. These represented ten parts that could break, yet he proposed to implant this Rube Goldberg device into a human being.

Another realm of privilege for doctors was sex. Many times I have seen doctors propositioning nurses before, during, and after surgery. I have heard many a surgeon tell a circulating nurse that the string holding up his scrub pants was loose, and would she please pull his greens up. The nurse, to accommodate him, would reach around and fondle his genitals. I have seen many a doctor position himself behind a nurse and run his hand under her dress. In one instance, a nurse screamed in protest and the operating-room supervisor, equally outraged, barred the doctor from doing elective surgery in her operating room for a month. But in many hospitals—judging by the number of similar happenings—not only would the nurse not protest, she would accept.

Unfortunately (for the nurses) most doctors are already married, though some behave more like single men. The public, perhaps as part of the Me Doctor Syndrome, expects more circumspect behavior from physicians. Yet I have noticed on numerous occasions the wide gap between expectation and reality. A well-known orthopedic surgeon once dined in New York City with me and a representative from my company's home office. Throughout the evening, the doctor kept saying, "Do you know any places around here where a guy can get laid?" He was not too subtle. Finally I told him there was a massage parlor in the next block, and he made some off-color comment about going there for dessert. During the rest of dinner, he was like a man obsessed. "I wonder what the place is like. What kind of girls do they have?" and so forth. When we paid the check, he was the first out of the seat. Jeff Wright, as I will call my friend, and I walked him down Third Avenue. Outside the establishment a hawker handed out flyers offering a free massage.

"How many girls do you have upstairs?" the doctor asked.

"We have seven girls working tonight."

"How much?"

"Fifty dollars." The doctor turned to me for a fifty-dollar "loan."

I gave it to him because he asked me to. Jeff and I sat in a bar next door waiting for the doctor. About twenty minutes later he came down, and, for the rest of the evening, regaled us with his adventure. Never have I heard anybody embellish more on the sex act, especially one that lasted less than twenty minutes. Finally I could endure no more, and Jeff and I escorted the doctor to his car.

I saw him several times during the next month because he ordered a considerable amount of equipment from me. One day, while I was talking to him in a hospital corridor, he said, "We must have dinner again soon." I assumed that he wanted me to spring for another fifty, although he never repaid the first loan.

Another time a resident who had no money and was sharing a room with another doctor asked to borrow the keys to my room at the Fairmount Hotel in San Francisco. We were attending the 1975 annual meeting of the American Academy of Orthopedic Surgeons. Orthopedists, like other doctors (or humans), prefer to hold their conventions in such idyllic locales as Las Vegas, New Orleans, Dorado Beach in Puerto Rico, or The Greenbriar, a grand hotel in West Virginia. The doctor in San Francisco had encountered a woman at the hotel bar. I thought her extremely unsavory, but he apparently did not, because he disappeared with her for an hour. A month later, he joked with me about how he had to take penicillin when he started having a burning sensation while urinating. At the same meeting a year earlier in Dallas (to illustrate the range of services performed for doctors) three other salesmen and I spent forty-five minutes extracting an elderly physician from a phone booth in the foyer of the main ballroom of the Hilton. Apparently he had gone in there for a quiet drink and had managed to wedge his body against the door. We carried him back to his hotel and left him to sober up in bed.

Still, these privileges and licenses are relatively minor compared to the cover-ups. Nurses, subscribing to the Me Doctor Syndrome, often cover for doctors by performing various chores they have overlooked. For example, I knew of one doctor who, after completing gall-bladder surgery, hurried back to office hours. He did not notice that one blood vessel in the patient's abdomen was still bleeding and covered the incision with a bandage. About an hour later, the operating-room supervisor called to say the patient was still bleeding despite pressure bandages and other efforts to stop the hemorrhage. Ordinarily, the recovery-room supervisor would have reported the problem, but this particular doctor had a hot temper, and nobody liked to deal with him except the OR supervisor.

The doctor's office was five minutes away by car, but instead of returning to the hospital to take care of his patient, he asked the OR supervisor how Mrs. X was doing.

"Is she awake?"

"No, but she's starting to come around," the nurse replied.

"Do me a favor," the surgeon said. "Clamp off the bleeder and throw a stitch into it for me."

And the nurse did. This incident strikes me as the epitome of neglect, because the patient was paying the doctor, not the nurse, to take primary care of her. The nurse did something she was not licensed or trained to do, and compounded that offense by covering for the doctor's laziness.

Altering operating-room reports was a far more serious form of cover-up. To my knowledge, I was never logged into surgery. The official records of the procedures I attended—with one exception when a nurse logged me in at one hospital as "Dr. MacKay"—never acknowledged my presence in the operating room. Yet these reports supposedly list everybody present. My omission from the list accorded that much more protection to the hospital, the doctors, and the staff.

The operating-room report itself is a vehicle for cover-up. After every procedure, the surgeon is supposed to dictate notes about the case. The report should be a warts-and-all account, but doctors understandably dictate with an eye on future malpractice suits. Nobody checks the records or contradicts the doctor's account. Consider the operating-room report in the Mirando case. Dr. Lipton claimed that Franklin Mirando had a hairline fracture of the femur. At one point in that procedure, I was looking at three, possibly four, splits in the bone. They were no hairline fractures, by anybody's account. But Lipton was not about to acknowledge that he had fractured the entire end of the patient's femur while removing an incorrectly placed prosthesis.

Lipton hoped that the patient would recover fully and that no disaster would develop later on.

Again, page two of the operating-room report of the total hip case described in Chapter 1 stated: "During the procedure on the trial run it was found that too great an anteversion had been obtained, and the final position seating was adequate, appropriate, and acceptable. The wound was then closed." The report fails to mention that the hip prosthesis had to be removed, that new cement was placed in the patient, and that a different prosthetic component was installed. Nor did the report mention that it took at least two hours just to remove the cement, or that Bill MacKay did it. A reader would think this was a normal, run-of-the-mill procedure when, in fact, it was a disaster. This operating-room report was inaccurate, incomplete, and so, I must assume, were many others.

TWELVE

BAD CASES

Long before the world learned in October 1977 that a medical-equipment salesman had performed surgery on Franklin Mirando's hip, my surgical work had gradually become known in the medical community of Long Island. In fact, about two weeks after that first total hip case, when Tom Merriman proposed sawing the patient's femur in half, I attended an orthopedic conference. Dr. Merriman displayed his X rays on the viewbox and described the case to the assembled doctors. To my surprise, the dozen or so surgeons present seemed totally aware of my role in helping Merriman and Kasik during that case. Merriman did not say in so many words that I had bailed him out, but it became apparent, judging by the comments and questions directed at me during the meeting, that word had gone out about my participation. The Chief of Surgery at one hospital said, "I hear you were involved in that long total hip case with Dr. Merriman." Another orthopedic surgeon told me, "Boy, I'm glad you guys got out of that case all right." And much later a surgeon whose actual name is Dr. Jim Murray told a *Newsday* reporter, "It was common knowledge that some surgeons wouldn't go into the operating room without Bill MacKay. . . . His knowledge of implants was tremendous."

Nor was knowledge of my activities confined to doctors. Nurses, OR supervisors, anesthesiologists, and other salesmen knew I frequented the operating room. Even hospital administrators were aware, because they had to authorize my presence. When one doctor invited me to observe a case, the assistant operating-room supervisor called the hospital administrator and obtained permission. No formal procedure existed, but I know that the administrator, whom I shall call Sam Donovan, fully understood and endorsed my activities. I learned of his awareness one time when I asked the assistant hospital administrator, Bill Root, I will name him, for authorization to replace a dermatome, which shaves off skin for grafting. A doctor had dropped the $900 instrument on the floor, and Root called in his boss to approve the purchase. When Donovan came in, he wore a light blue shirt, no tie, and a pair of Scotch plaid pants. I remember thinking, "Is this a hospital or a country club?" He looked like he was ready for eighteen holes at St. Andrews.

Donovan inspected the dermatome: "Were you there when it happened? You're there for all our major orthopedic cases, right?"

"Yes, sir," I said.

On another occasion, I made an emergency delivery to the operating-room supervisor. She had needed a two-inch Jewett nail in a hurry, and I took it directly to her, violating Donovan's rule that salesmen inform him when they entered the hospital. When she called his office for a purchase order, he must have asked whether I was there, because I heard her say, "Yes, he is." Pause. "Well," she said, "this is an emergency. I needed the nail right away and told him to come directly to me." Pause. "Hey," she said, "whenever we've got a total hip case, I want him in the operating room with the doctors!"

Several times thereafter, Sam Donovan sat down with me and inquired about the quality of total hip procedures in his hospital. Bill Root was present on one occasion when Donovan asked why things went wrong during total hip procedures. Donovan had a copy of the operating-room schedule on his desk each day. If a major orthopedic case was scheduled, he knew I would be there. He frequently saw me enter the hospital coffee shop in the presence of surgeons, and in full view of everybody, with blood all over my greens. Donovan and Root were sitting in the coffee shop one day as a surgeon and I walked in after a case. They motioned us to sit at their table. Although we wore lab coats over our greens, which is acceptable attire in a hospital eatery, it was obvious where we had been because our foot covers were bloodied. That day Donovan asked me, "How did the case go?" I said, "Pretty good. We knocked it out in an hour and a half." (This was not a play on words.) In other words, Sam Donovan was fully aware that I frequented his operating rooms, that I assisted surgeons and touched patients. He never actually saw me operate, but he knew what I was doing and encouraged my doing it.

Meanwhile, as a result of my surgical activities, sales were soaring. When competitors tried to sell a product, many doctors would say, "I buy from MacKay. He takes care of us." Before long, it became known in the industry that salesmen need not apply in some areas of Long Island. I had it locked up, especially after I became distributor for an orthopedic-device company. One reason business boomed is that other salesmen, who also scrubbed in with doctors, started bringing me cases they could not handle. They received full credit for selling the equipment used in the procedure and full credit for providing what the surgeon needed—me. This arrangement benefited me as well. It relieved the salesmen who worked for me so they could be out selling and insured that they did not bungle any cases.

After I started my distributorship, I reviewed surgical techniques with my salesmen at night, just as Harry Fontaine once did with me. Part of my function as sales manager included teaching them all I could, for handiness in the operating room had proved an undisputed boon to sales. Three of my salesmen did their share of surgery. George Schott, of craniotomy fame, specialized in the neuro division of MacKay and Company, another salesman specialized in trauma, a third specialized in playing golf with doctors, and I specialized in total joints. Only George has been asked to testify as of this writing, so I see no reason to bring the surgical expertise of the others to the foreground.

As my own exploits became known, doctors started coming to me to discuss their cases, particularly the difficult ones. By spring 1975, even before the Mirando case, I was in great demand because many surgeons who once invited me into surgery *in case* they ran into problems now consulted me *because* they anticipated problems. I became part of the surgical team at a number of hospitals. Doctors approached me not primarily about the products I was selling but about the surgical problems of implanting those products. Some doctors even telephoned and literally pleaded with me to come into surgery with them. An orthopedic surgeon called me one day and asked me to attend his first total hip procedure. I declined because he was using my competitor's products and their make of hip, and I then represented another firm. Before hanging up the phone, however, I spent an hour explaining every detail of the procedure to him. Earlier that day he had called my wife and told her he needed me there because I was the best in the business. The point was not that I was helping doctors during surgery, but the extent to which I was helping them.

My surgical activities caused one surgeon to warn me, on more than one occasion, about getting involved with the wrong kind of surgeons, and two in particular. "Those guys are going to get into trouble," he predicted.

"What do you mean?"

"I mean somebody's going to get crippled or die. I mean you're going to get caught!"

Nor was he the only surgeon who warned me. There are times when I wish I had heeded their advice. On the other hand, if I had, my opportunities to operate would have been fewer. As matters stood, my experiences with surgeons, good and bad, ranged from head to toe, or, more precisely, ankle.

Starting with the head, I was once called to a hospital on Long Island by the central supply supervisor of the department which distributes and purchases all surgical equipment. After I arrived, he told me that a neurosurgeon was having problems with a Hall II air driver my company distributed. This instrument is used to saw off the skull during a craniotomy. When I arrived at the hospital, the supply supervisor—call him Fred—seemed annoyed. "A neurosurgeon is doing the case right now, and he's breaking blades like crazy. At $33 a blade, we're going to go broke. Can you go talk to him?" He telephoned the operating-room supervisor and told her that Mr. MacKay was coming in to check the instrument.

The OR supervisor told me to scrub and escorted me to the doctor's lounge. When I entered the operating room, I saw a surgeon I had never met before holding the air driver and looking extremely frustrated.

"I'm from the manufacturer," I said, "and you're using our air driver. Is there anything I can do to help?"

"Yes, the goddam thing doesn't work. It's no good."

"Doctor, maybe you're holding the blade wrong. Show me how you're using it."

He demonstrated his technique, which reminded me of the scene from the craniotomy I had observed with George Schott several years earlier. This surgeon was holding the air driver as if he were trying to cut the top off a pumpkin.

"You shouldn't lean that far, Doctor. That's why the blade is getting stuck. You are supposed to hold it directly at right angles to the skull." He then informed me that he had done nine hundred (or some equally implausible number) of similar procedures in Vietnam. "Well, you are doing this one wrong," I said, and pointed out that five drill bits already were broken in the patient's skull. For several minutes silence reigned. Then he said, "Come over here and show me."

He did not bother to inquire whether I had done craniotomies before. (I had not.) He did not ask my name. Knowing only that I sold an air driver he could not operate, he let me take the instrument and cut into his patient's skull. I held the instrument perpendicular to the skull and, in less than two minutes, removed the skull cap without breaking any more drill bits. I handed the instrument back to the doctor.

"When you hold it at a right angle, the blades don't break."

"Uh, yeah, I see what you mean."

He gazed at the broken blades now displayed atop the membrane that separates the skull from the brain.

"Well, I'll be seeing you," I said, and walked out of the room. Later I told Fred that this surgeon would keep popping blades as long as he held the air driver at the wrong angle.

"What if he keeps doing it?" Fred asked.

"If I were you," I said, "I would order a dozen more blades."

A similar but somewhat gentler instrument was a key character in a mastoid case I once assisted in. This turbine-driven, nitrogen-powered air drill is a highly sophisticated instrument that operates at 130,000 rpm. The hospital had just purchased a Hall II from me for about $1000. One day the operating-room supervisor asked me to demonstrate it to an ENT (ear-nose-throat) surgeon. He was planning mastoid surgery, and wanted somebody there who was familiar with the instrument. I did not want to attend the case, because I did no business with eye, ear, nose, and throat surgeons, nor did I have interest or experience in that specialty. But it was a command performance, and I went.

Occasionally a patient develops a middle ear infection which spreads to the mastoid bone, which is just behind the ear. The surgeon corrects the problem by removing diseased tissue. In the operating room it became apparent that the doctor was having trouble drilling through the mastoid bone. He asked what was wrong, and I showed him. "Okay, let me try it again," he said. He revved the motor all the way to 130,000 rpm and resumed drilling. I noticed that he leaned on the drill and was very heavy-handed. The next thing I knew, blood was gushing out of the patient four feet into the air. He apparently had hit a large artery, judging from the force of the bleeding. It looked like a small oil-well gusher.

"My God," he said, "what are we going to do?"

"Doctor," I said, "the first thing we do is put a piece of cotton over the bleeder."

We grabbed cotton sponges and anything else that might stop the bleeding, but the flow was so heavy we had to change sponges every five seconds. Finally I wrapped my right thumb in a piece of cotton gauze and shoved it against the hole where the blood was gushing out. As the bleeding came under control, the tension in the room relaxed, the doctor regained his composure, and called in a general surgeon to help him sew up the blood vessel. At that point I left, thus ending my participation in a mastoid case.

A doctor in the Bronx once told me he intended to implant a total elbow prosthesis in a patient, and invited me to his office to show him the Pritchard-Walker Mark II elbow. I also showed him a movie on how to implant it. Total elbows were relatively new at the time, and only a few surgeons in the New York area had implanted them. This surgeon—Dr. Frank Iseman I will call him—had never done a total elbow before, although he had done total hips and other implants. He seemed to think the elbow would be no problem.

"Fine, Doctor, when's the case?"

"A week from tomorrow."

The next day, Dr. Iseman left word that he wanted to see the movie again. That weekend we watched the film four more times at his home. "I've got this thing down cold," he declared. "There will be no problem." The patient, he explained, had broken his elbow previously. It was fused in a flexed position, and the arm had little function.

On the day surgery was scheduled, I had a blockbuster head cold. I went to the hospital anyway, planning to make sales calls.

"I've got a hell of a cold," I told Dr. Iseman. "Maybe I shouldn't be in on the case."

"No, no," he said, "I want you there. Wear two masks."

I relented, though later I wished I had not. About forty-five minutes into the case, Dr. Iseman, while looking for the medullary canal, popped off a condyle, a knob at the elbow end of the humerus or upper arm bone. Considering his technique for locating the canal, the damage might have been worse. He had used an air driver at full power as a probe, instead of a taper reamer or some gentler instrument. In the process, he destroyed a piece of bone the size of a thumb joint that was to serve as anchorage for the new prosthesis.

Dr. Iseman fussed around with the elbow for several minutes, then—realizing he had bitten (or drilled) off more than he could handle—announced his solution. "I'm going to give this patient a hanging arm instead of an implant." He intended to pull a flap of muscle over the ends of the bone, to prevent the surfaces from rubbing against one another, and sew up the incision. A hanging arm, which is comparable to a hanging hip, is usually reserved for elderly patients to relieve pain caused by arthritis. But this was a young man who would never be able to bend or raise his arm. It would, in effect, be useless.

The case was not yet over. From the doctor's lounge, I then heard Dr. Iseman telephone the patient's wife, who was out in the lobby, rather than confront her face-to-face. In broken Spanish, he said, "Maria, Maria, we tried to do the elbow, but the bone was just too small. He's got a free arm now." As I listened to him "console" her in phony Spanish, I remember thinking, "This guy is about as Puerto Rican as I am, and he's trying to convince this woman that he's one of her people. And he just ruined her husband's elbow."

On another occasion in the spring of 1977, a scoliosis surgeon insisted (and I do mean _insisted,_ because he phoned me numerous times) that I watch him operate on a patient with scoliosis. This disease causes the spine to curve into an S. In severe cases one shoulder might, from the front view, be four inches lower than the other. A related disease, kyphosis, causes the spine to curve from front to back. Scoliosis attacks predominantly adolescent girls. The skeletal disorder does not, in itself, kill its victims, but it can put so much stress on the internal anatomy—compressing the lungs, heart, and liver and causing these organs to malfunction for lack of space—that untreated victims often die. The cure for this terrible affliction is a special body brace, in which the patient is sometimes imprisoned for years. Even with surgery, a victim usually must live in a cast for eight months.

In scoliosis surgery, the doctor inserts a steel rod inside the patient's body to force the spine into a straight line. The doctor who insisted that I watch this procedure—I will call him Doctor Mark Avison—told me to meet him around eight in the morning. When I arrived, he said, "Let me show you around first. I have a lot of patients in the hospital right now. I'm one of this hospital's biggest supporters." He led me to a pavilion where most of his patients were hospitalized. As we moved from bed to bed, he told one and all, "This is Dr. MacKay." "Dr. MacKay is working with me today." "Dr. MacKay wanted to come in and observe a scoliosis case." That day I saw teen-age girls with braces and casts extending from their pubic areas to their necks. They were pretty girls, and I found myself feeling sorry for them because they must have felt miserable lying there with deformed backs, surrounded by spectators. Dr. Avison finally tired of making rounds and led me to the doctor's lounge, where we put on scrub suits. He then introduced me to the operating-room supervisor: "This is Dr. MacKay, he's going to be in surgery with me today." I had been making sales calls at her office for years, but he never bothered to ask if I knew her. We looked at one another and neither of us said a word. Nurses have the most marvelously inscrutable faces.

As we entered the operating room of this eminent teaching institution, I saw the patient, a fifteen-year-old girl, lying stomach down in a bent position on the operating table. Two residents had already opened her back with an incision nearly eighteen inches long by six inches wide. All along the opening, Weitlaner retractors were in place. There must have been twelve of these scissorlike instruments spreading the incision.

It was impossible to tell how long our late arrival had delayed the operation. As Dr. Avison made his grand entrance, the atmosphere in the room became hushed, reverential. A resident stood at each side of the table and a scrub technician—who was not a registered nurse—stood on the patient's right. Had I been able to plug speakers into the residents' heads, I am sure I would have heard them playing "Hail to the Chief!"

The chief took a sharp, razorlike gouge and began cutting small pieces of bone from the chain of vertebrae that form the spinal column. He handed the pieces to a resident, who placed them in a stainless-steel specimen bowl and, with a scissors, cut them into slivers the size of matchsticks. They would be used later to fuse the spine. Removing the bone helped make the spine more supple and easy to straighten. Meanwhile, the other resident injected coagulant with a huge 50cc syringe into the incision to slow the bleeding. After Dr. Avison had removed two dozen bone chips, he took two hooks and attached them to each end of the spine. He then took a ratchet device called an outrigger, attached it between the two hooks, turned the crank, and expanded it to stretch the spine into a straight line.

As I watched this mechanical monstrosity, I realized that this girl was lucky. Sometimes the patient is kept awake and given a local anesthetic so that she can wiggle her toes to show the surgeon that her spine is not injured. When Dr. Avison achieved the degree of straightness he wanted, he replaced the outrigger with a stainless surgical-steel rod measuring one and a half feet. He attached the bottom hook, then slid the top hook, notch by notch, up a series of ratchets. Finally, he placed a washer below the top hook to keep it from sliding back down.

At this point, Dr. Avison looked like Napoleon after he had crowned himself Emperor. He announced, "Great case! What do you think of that, Bill? A scoliosis case in one hour!" With that he told the residents, "Okay, close her up. I'll speak to her later this afternoon." And he sailed out of the room, bidding me to follow in his wake.

"Who," I thought, "does he think he's kidding?" It must have taken thirty minutes at least to open this patient up and strip the spine of muscles, ligaments, and tendons. Just because this surgeon removed some bone and implanted two hooks and a rod did not mean the case was finished. Indeed, another forty-five minutes' work remained, because the fusion had not yet been done. All those little matchsticks of bone were not yet placed lengthwise along the spinal column so they could, in six months' time, grow together and weld the spine in its new, straightened position. Packing them into place may not have been difficult, but the ultimate success of the operation depended upon getting a good graft. The rod, which Dr. Avison implanted with such ceremony, is no more than a temporary traction device that is often removed after the spine fuses.

But Dr. Avison elected to leave that girl with an eighteen-by-six-inch gap in her back. He chose to abandon her before the fusion was done. What would have prevented one of those residents, while fusing the spine, from making an error that might have damaged the spinal cord or endangered her life? What, I thought, about her parents, who entrusted their daughter to this man?

My final comment is that Dr. Avison settled for a fifty percent reduction in spinal curvature. Yet he could have achieved a straighter back had he put more tension on the rod, for which it was designed. He frequently settled for seventy to eighty percent reduction in curvature, rather than try for ninety to ninety-five percent or a nearly perfect spine. This he did, in my opinion, because he feared that applying more tension might break the rod six months or two years hence and cause a malpractice suit. This may be prudent, defensive medicine, but it places the doctor's interests ahead of the patient's.

The scoliosis case was memorable because I witnessed so few of them. I attended many hip cases, but one was unusual because I went to the hospital under police escort. One Good Friday I sat at my desk anticipating a three-day weekend with my wife and children in Connecticut. Meanwhile, at a hospital twenty miles away, an attending surgeon and three residents were implanting a total hip prosthesis. As I was soon to learn, they cemented in the plastic cup, drilled out the femur, and did a trial reduction with a test prosthesis. While the residents were mixing the cement, the attending surgeon left to do office hours. Before the residents could position the permanent prosthesis, the cement hardened in the femur. The operating-room supervisor, at this point, called my office, told me a hip prosthesis was stuck halfway in a patient's femur, and asked me to bring a cement-removal set over right away. This is a set of medullary reamers or drills of varying diameters, plus some osteotomes used to chisel and pulverize the cement. I agreed to deliver the instruments to the hospital in twenty minutes. As I was driving along the Grand Central Parkway, I spotted a policeman, stopped and asked him to escort me, since I planned to be driving at about eighty miles an hour. When I arrived in this spectacular fashion at the hospital, the OR supervisor asked me to familiarize the three residents with the cement-removal instruments.

When I entered the operating room, I discovered that they were foreigners. Their English was hard to understand, although they seemed to understand me well enough. The room was in total chaos. They were chipping pieces off the femur and destroying the top end as they tried to remove the cement. One resident was saying, "Let's do this." Another would say, "No, let's do that." It reminded me of a sinking ship with the crew running around the decks. I surveyed the scene and decided not to get wet.

"Hold it," I said. "Everybody stop what you're doing and look at the clock. It is three o'clock, and we're going to be here another hour and a half, no more, no less. So let's stop all this helter-skelter and start taking our time." I ordered an air driver and nine-sixty-fourth-inch bit from the circulating nurse, who hooked it to the nitrogen tank. As I pulverized the cement, the three residents looked abashed, because I made the job look so easy. Fifteen minutes later I finished removing the cement.

"Gentlemen," I said, "mix a new batch of cement, put in the prosthesis, and close the patient up." With that, I walked out, removed my mask and scrub suit, and took off for Connecticut.

The attending surgeon, in my opinion, used poor judgment leaving the cast to those residents. He might have felt they were perfectly capable, but it is customary to stay in the operating room until the case ends. However, this was a service patient, which may explain the medical care he received. The sequel to this case was that the following Monday one of my salesmen went to the hospital, where the same attending surgeon told him the reason the prosthesis did not fit (and, by implication, the reason the cement hardened before it could be positioned properly) was that my company had provided a trial prosthesis different in size from the permanent one. This accusation enraged me. I immediately went to the hospital and showed the Chief of Orthopedics and the attending surgeon that the two prostheses were, to the centimeter, the same. If anybody was at fault, I told them, it was the attending surgeon, who should have remained in the OR to make sure everything fit. This episode was, from start to finish, a cover-your-ass operation.

Another debacle involved a knee case. Dr. John Perth, as I call him, was planning his first total knee procedure, and asked whether I had a movie about the Marmor knee prosthesis that we sold. Several days later I took the movie to the doctor's lounge, where we watched it together several times. Apparently he felt confident that he could install the knee, because he did not invite me to scrub for the case. But he did ask me to be there.

On the morning of surgery, I watched Perth fashion beds in the distal end of the femur. An assistant surgeon mixed methylmethacrylate, and Perth packed it into the bone. But instead of placing the front of the prosthesis in the front, he put it in backward. Meanwhile, the cement had hardened. At that moment I was not paying close attention to the procedure. Suddenly I heard him exclaim that the knee was in backward.

"That's okay, we can knock the thing out and put a new one in," I said.

"What are we going to do with all the cement?" he cried.

"Don't worry about it," I said.

I left the room, at his request, to scrub. When I returned, I took a mallet and tapped an osteotome against the implant. After several minutes, I managed to pry it loose. We both picked away at the hardened cement, and the assistant surgeon mixed up a new batch.

"Do you want me to put the prosthesis in for you?" I asked.

"Yes, put it in," Perth said. "That way, we'll know it's in right."

I was chuckling to myself as I packed cement into the slots Perth had drilled. I inserted both parts of the prosthesis, and stepped back so Perth could sew up the knee.

Farther down the leg, a doctor I will call George Mundy, who planned to implant a total ankle, once called me to detail a Mayo-type ankle. It is a boxlike structure, with a plastic component that is cemented into the lower end of the tibia. A steel component is implanted in the talar, the bone between the heel and tibia and the largest bone in the foot. The prosthesis is installed much like a total knee, with considerable bone carving to create a bed to fit the device. I had scrubbed with this surgeon before and, as usual, he asked me to observe the case. As the operation began, Dr. Mundy made a curvilinear or "lazy S" skin incision down the midline of the ankle. He then located the major tendons in the area and tied two matching pieces of suture to each tendon, using different styles of sutures so he would know which ends to reconnect. Then he cut each tendon with a scissors. They snapped like rubber bands out of sight, retrievable only by the sutures which dangled like strings from deep inside the leg.

With an osteotome, Dr. Mundy began chiseling the tibia, and I began chatting with the circulating nurse (which made me guilty of the same bad habit I have criticized doctors for). Several minutes later, I noticed that he had cut too much bone from the talar and had broken off part of the tibia, which is part of the supporting wall for the implant. He had made such a mess that it

130

was impossible to repair the bone or implant a total ankle that would have any chance of success. As soon as Dr. Mundy broke off the tibia, I went out and scrubbed. I knew what was coming. When I returned, he was fingering the tibial prosthesis as if he still intended to use it.

"Doctor," I said, "I think you had better do a fusion."

"I'm doing a total ankle."

"You don't have a choice any more between a total or fused ankle," I insisted. "The prosthesis will never hold with this much tibia missing. You will have to fuse the ankle."

At this point he realized that an implant would be impossible, and asked me to help him.

I had never fused an ankle, although I had read about and seen diagrams of the procedure. Essentially, the surgeon planes off the tibia and talar so that they fit against each other and places as many bone chips as are available in between. It is essential to have healthy, bleeding bones so that they will later grow together. Dr. Mundy took a device called a Charnley arthrodesis clamp. It is an eight-and-a-half-inch square whose most arresting features are two three-sixteenth-inch diameter Steinmann pins that pierce the shin and ankle. Dr. Mundy drilled a hole through the patient's tibia about six inches above the ankle and another hole through the talar. He inserted the Steinmann pins, and I helped attach and tighten the clamps at the sides. This device totally immobilizes the ankle while the two bones fuse together. The patient lies in bed in a plaster cast for six weeks, then graduates to a short leg cast for another four weeks or longer. Although the patient loses some motion in the ankle, he goes home with a pain-free joint and the assurance that the ankle will need no further surgery.

There are other problems with these new artificial joints. With the possible exception of the total hip, frequently they do not work, nor do they last. A total ankle might function twelve months at most. Total knees also have multitudes of failures, including infection, loosening, and pain. My mother had her first total knee implanted in 1972. She had her second knee implanted in 1975. Now that one is beginning to fail, which means her knee will have to be fused. God willing, when they open her up, they will not infect her and have to amputate her leg, because every time a surgeon reoperates on the same area, the likelihood of infection and other complications increases.

Even total hips, which work very well, do not last forever.

Yet a surgeon tells a patient, "With this new hip you will be able to walk. Your swelling will disappear, and so will the pain." He neglects to mention that the hip will last only fifteen years. Thus a fifty-five-year-old total hip patient will likely need another at age seventy. At age seventy, he will not withstand surgery as well as at age fifty-five.

Artificial knees, elbows, and ankles remain unproven for the long haul, and the only way doctors can perfect them is by putting them in patients. Surgeons will continue to do this, unhampered by government regulation. And nonpaying service patients will continue to serve as guinea pigs because they are in total awe of doctors and are too old, too uneducated, and too poor to fight back when things go wrong.

A case in point: A surgeon on the South Shore area—Dr. Richard Furgurson, I will call him—heard that my firm had just introduced a new total ankle. When I brought the prosthesis to Dr. Furgurson's office, he rang for his secretary: "Get me the X rays on Mr. Z. I want to implant one of these ankles, and this guy is a beautiful candidate." The surgeon had planned to fuse this patient's ankle, which was pained and crippled with arthritis. But now he was willing to implant a new device because a salesman had dropped it in his lap.

I, the salesman, sold these devices even though they were unperfected. In some instances I would point out this fact, and the doctor would reply, "I realize that, but I've got to do something for this patient now." More often, I rationalized my role by telling myself: "As long as they're going to implant an ankle, it might as well be the one I sell."

So Dr. Furgurson, having bought my ankle, asked me to detail the case to him, since he had never done one before. He also invited me to attend the case and—in a request that had become familiar—asked me to take photographs of the proce-dure. A week later when I arrived in the operating room, film and camera in hand, he acted as if he had done the procedure fifteen times. "We can do this ankle in an hour. It shouldn't be any problem at all," he said.

I was not scrubbed during the early part of the case because I was busy snapping pictures. Suddenly I noticed that Dr. Furgur-son, who had cemented in the talar component, was having trouble making the tibial or upper half of the implant bond to the bone. The cement had hardened, but the prosthesis was loose and wobbly. Dr. Furgurson removed the tibial component, chipped out the cement, and tried again. Same result. Then he asked me to try. But the tibia was bleeding so profusely that the cement would not cure properly and I could not get proper fixation. Finally I suggested that Dr. Furgurson reapply a tourniquet around the tibia and pack the upper area with bone wax to stop the bleeding long enough to implant the tibial component correctly. But he was not interested. "I think I've got it now," he said, as the prosthesis wiggled in his hand. I protested and told him it was still loose.

"Nah, I'm going to close up. I've fooled with this thing long enough."

"In that case, Doctor," I said, "you won't be needing me any more," and I left. The patient left with a wobbly ankle which, I am sure, soon became painful and nonfunctional. But the doctor was too busy to bother doing it right. I refused to scrub with Dr. Furgurson again.

On several occasions, I was a victim of surgical mishaps. Once I was holding a retractor in a knee incision while the surgeon chiseled the femur with an osteotome. He glanced at the assistant surgeon for a moment while his mallet was coming down. It struck an osteotome, and it slipped off the side of the bone and drove deep into the top of my hand. The surgeon was too engrossed in conversation to realize what happened until I yelled in pain that he had cut my hand. It was bleeding so heavily that I went to the emergency room, where they put three stitches in it. My participation in the case thus ended, but the scar on my hand lingers on.

Another misadventure involved a total hip procedure. Little suspecting what was about to happen, I brought the instruments to the hospital and gave an in-service training program to the operating-room nurses. The surgeon—Dr. Ralph Oblensky I will call him—did not review the case with me, even though he had never done a Charnley total hip before. Still, from talking to him, he seemed familiar with the procedure. The operating-room supervisor asked me to scrub, for the usual reason: to be sure the nurses knew which instruments to hand the doctors.

Several days later, I joined the two assistant surgeons around the operating table in Nassau County. One of them had witnessed several total hip cases, the other had never seen one. As the case started, Dr. Oblensky, who thought he knew all about the procedure, took more than an hour to drape the unconscious patient. Usually this takes about fifteen minutes. Next he could not find the greater trochanter, which is the point of reference for making the initial incision. I couldn't believe what I was seeing. Finally the other surgeon helped Dr. Oblensky find the greater trochanter, and the latter proceeded to open the hip. Dr. Oblensky asked me for the U-shaped initial-incision retractor. I handed it to him in the proper position. He then put it in the patient upside down. When I brought this to his attention, he gave me a baleful look and left the retractor upside down. Before long, he discovered that he could not place his hand inside the patient's hip because the retractor was in the way. He reinserted it properly with the open end of the U facing the patient's head.

Next he prepared to cut the neck of the femur. I suggested using a Gigli saw. "I've seen it done with an osteotome," he said, and selected one of the largest ones on the instrument table. When the scrub nurse handed it to him, he smashed it into the neck of the femur, severing it, not from the sharpness of the osteotome but from the force of the impact. Next he took a Meyerding bone skid, which looks like a shoehorn, and slid it between the acetabulum and femoral head to break the suction between the two. But he jammed it in so hard that it perforated the floor of the acetabulum. To correct the damage, Dr. Oblensky had to place wire mesh over the perforation so bone cement would not leak through the acetabulum and into the patient's pelvis.

He then inserted the acetabular cup, inclining it too far toward the floor. I told him that this was incorrect. Having become more receptive to my suggestions by now, he pulled it out, removed the cement, and inserted new wire mesh. At this point he said, "Since you have seen so many Charnley procedures, would you position the cup in the acetabulum?" As usual, I complied.

When it came time to ream the femoral canal, Dr. Oblensky took a standard bone rasp (the wrong instrument for the job) and used so much force driving it into the opening that it pierced the femur. Now he had a pea-sized hole in the side of the femur, which he repaired by holding his finger over it while I put in cement and positioned the femoral prosthesis.

Dr. Oblensky then asked me to drill three holes in the greater trochanter for the wires that would reattach it to the femur. But when he began threading the eighteen-gauge wire through the holes, he ran it through the tip of my left index finger, which was holding the greater trochanter against the femur as a person would hold a knot being tied around a package. Before I could feel the full impact of pain, Dr. Oblensky snapped the wire tight. My finger was securely attached to the patient's greater trochanter. I screamed in agony. He looked at me with surprise and loosened the wire but did not release it. I explained that he had driven the wire through my finger and it was attached to the patient.

"Oh, it's probably only your glove," he said, brushing off my complaint.

"No, Doctor, it is my finger!" To emphasize my point, I called him a "dumb bastard." Only after I had cussed him out was he convinced that he had to restring the wire.

After he pulled the wire back out, my finger was bleeding profusely into my glove and into the patient. It made us, as the Indians say, blood brother and sister. The patient was full of intravenous antibiotics. But I was not. The chance of my being infected was great. I stayed long enough to help Dr. Oblensky tighten the knots on the wire, and left the operating room, my finger throbbing in pain. Out in the hallway, the operating-room supervisor said, "Are you cut?"

"Yes, he ran the wire through my finger and attached me to the patient."

"Oh, God!" she said, "we've got to get you a shot."

She called the emergency room. A nurse came running with a syringe in her hand, pushed up the sleeve of my scrub suit, and plunged the needle into my arm. I have no idea what she injected.

"When's the last time you had a tetanus shot?" she asked.

"It's been a while."

She produced another syringe from her pocket and blasted the same arm without even asking whether I was allergic to the medication. But she was, I am sure, doing her best.

About thirty minutes later, Dr. Oblensky found me recuperating near the operating-room supervisor's desk.

"Boy, that was great," he said. "We've got to do more of these. The patient's got a good range of motion, and she's going to be fine."

I remember sitting there, looking up at this doctor, absolutely speechless. I never scrubbed with him again.

An interesting postscript is that Dr. Oblensky told one of my salesmen how deplorable he thought the Mirando situation was, and how he would never let a salesman touch one of *his* patients. But I wouldn't let him cut my toenails. My souvenirs of working with him are the preoperative and postoperative X rays, the scar on my finger, and the knowledge that it was probably the most fouled-up case I ever witnessed.

THIRTEEN
GOOD CASES

People often say, "It's not so bad that MacKay did surgery as long as a doctor supervised it." But what about the times when a surgeon said, "Here, you do it!" Were these instances supervision or were they default? I would argue the latter.

One of my salesmen once asked me to prepare him for a Marmor total knee case with a surgeon I shall call Dr. Stuart Jehle, in the Bronx. I reviewed the procedure with the salesman several times, but he did not seem to grasp it. Finally he asked me to attend in his place. I visited Dr. Jehle and showed him the knee. It has two basic features, both of which bear out the unkind words I wrote about artificial implants earlier. The procedure does not require the intricate bone carving of the Geometric and other such knees. Secondly, the prosthesis comes not in two, but four, parts! The femoral portion consists of two convex metal components, each cemented into a trough the surgeon grinds in the two condyles at the lower end of the femur. The tibial portion consists of two half-moon-shaped plastic pieces, inserted into a scooped-out area atop the tibia and bordered by a small retaining wall of bone. The net result is a knee that is barely attached and highly unstable. My mother's first artificial knee, which lasted three years, was of this type. During the early 1970s, this knee

137

was touted as the greatest ever invented. The real reason for its popularity, however, was that it was easy to insert and required little technical skill on the part of the surgeon. Thus I found myself in league with Dr. Jehle, who had never done a total knee before.

On the morning of surgery he made the opening incision, then asked, "Should I do the femoral component or the tibial component first?"

"My God," I thought, "this surgeon doesn't know which way he's going."

"We do the femoral component first," I said. He took a Hall II air drill—the same 130,000-rpm model that ripped into an artery in the mastoid case—and plunged it into the lower end of the femur.

"Doctor, take your time," I said.

"Have you used one of these before?" he asked.

"Yes, I use them all the time." I showed him how to draw a centering line with a methylene blue marker down each femoral condyle. "Now, Doctor, we take the air drill and grind right down the lines I've drawn." The next thing I knew, he was mixing bone cement and I was putting it into the slots I had drilled. I looked at him, but he made no move to reclaim his place. So I asked the scrub nurse for the femoral prosthesis and inserted it. The lower-leg bone, the tibia, needed to be drilled. I drilled it. The tibial prosthesis needed to be cemented in place. I cemented it. In essence, I implanted the knee. All Doctor Jehle did was make the initial incision, put in Hemovac drains, mix cement, and stitch up the incision.

This kind of thing was happening with increasing frequency. In the evening my telephone would ring: "This is Doctor X. I'd like you to come in on a case with me." "This is Dr. Y. Can you be there Tuesday?" "This is Doctor Z's secretary and. . . ." Had I been paid $500 per case, I would have earned $40,000 a year and still not have charged for all the cases I was involved in. As it was, I never received a penny for doing surgery, nor should I have.

One of the most dramatic examples of a case in which I did most of the work occurred in the spring of 1975. A colleague who worked for my manufacturer in a New England state asked me to discuss a Charnley total hip procedure with a doctor who practiced in his territory. Because of my friendship with this salesman, I agreed. The following Thursday afternoon I drove up to meet the doctor in his office. He was a tall, gray-haired, distinguished-looking man, the kind who appears on television in a white lab coat to sell nasal decongestants or tell people to quit smoking. After fifteen minutes of conversation, it was apparent that this doctor (I will call him Dr. Bernard Seline) knew very little about the hip area, and even less about the prosthesis he intended to implant. We talked about the case over dinner and returned to his office to review X rays once again. With special red and yellow crayons I always carry in my coat pocket, I marked on the film where the surgeon should cut the femoral neck and the greater trochanter. This particular patient had a very shallow acetabulum, so I suggested that Dr. Seline fashion a deeper one by cutting some bone from the discarded femoral head and attach it with bone screws to create a lip for the acetabulum. As I talked to Dr. Seline, I could see that he understood my words but was not relating my explanation to the case at hand. I finally gave up and we drank sherry until around 11 P.M. Not until I was walking out the door did Dr. Seline tell me that the case was scheduled for the following Monday. Almost offhandedly, he asked, "Would you like to come and see the case?" I recall wondering, "Is he asking me or telling me?" I knew that my friend wanted me to scrub in, so I agreed.

The following Monday morning the alarm clock went off at the ungodly hour of 4:30 A.M., but I arose with the enthusiasm I usually reserved for Saturdays and drove up the New England Thruway. I arrived at the hospital on time and reported to the operating room, where the head nurse said, "Oh, Dr. MacKay, we've been expecting you. Dr. Seline said you'd be here, and I just wanted to ask what other hospitals you work at."

I named a couple of hospitals on Long Island. But I never told her I was a doctor, despite the obvious inference of my silence. I could see that she had been told—and not by me—that I was a doctor.

About five minutes later, Dr. Seline arrived and shook my hand: "Good morning, Dr. MacKay!" I then realized that his hospital disapproved of bringing salesmen into the operating room, hence the masquerade. We went to the doctor's lounge and put on surgical greens. Dr. Seline then introduced me to the assistant surgeon, who was about thirty-two years old. He had never seen a total hip either—or, if he had, he did not mention it. Dr. Seline made the initial skin incision using a standard Charnley approach. As soon as he exposed the hip capsule, he turned to me and said, "Dr. MacKay, would you please look at this?" I walked around the table and peered into the hip cavity. "Where do you think I should cut the femoral neck?" he asked. With my index finger, I pointed to the spot. He snaked a Gigli around the femur. But instead of sawing as I had suggested, he cut straight up and down, so that the angle was wrong. I pointed this out, and Dr. Seline asked how he should change it. "Let's bring the angle out toward the lateral aspect of the tip of the. . . ."

Dr. Seline stopped me in midsentence, handed me the Gigli saw, and, at that moment, he became the assistant and I became the surgeon. I reangled the femur, removed the greater trochanter, and reamed the acetabulum. The patient had a clean hip, that is, a hip which had never been operated upon before, but it was very arthritic. In addition, she had a congenital condition which caused her acetabulum to be very shallow. As I had recommended earlier, I cut a slightly curved piece off the femoral head, filed it, and attached it with large cortical bone screws to create a lip around the acetabulum and make it deeper. I cemented in the cup, reamed the femoral canal, and inserted the prosthesis. I then fastened the greater trochanter to the femur. When at last I looked up from my work, I told the assistant surgeon: "Doctor, why don't you close up the patient for me? My back is bothering me a bit." And I stepped back while he sewed up the patient.

About twenty minutes later, in the doctor's lounge, Dr. Seline told me, "Bill, that was marvelous. This woman has a good, stable hip now. I don't know how to thank you." As I was leaving the surgical area, the head nurse came up and said, "Dr. MacKay, I wasn't in the room, but I understand the case went very well. We really appreciate the time and effort you took to come here."

Everything about the experience proved rewarding. To this day I believe that Dr. Seline had no intention of doing that total hip. Perhaps our conversation the previous Thursday, or what he had previously heard about me, made this doctor intent upon having me present. I did everything except open and close the patient and cut the femoral head the wrong way. Other than that problem, everything went extremely well.

On the other hand, I saw many cases where surgeons should have won prizes for their work. One day in late spring, 1975, I received a message from a surgeon who lived just over the George Washington Bridge in New Jersey. It turned out I had met him at several orthopedic conferences. He planned to implant a new T-28 total hip and asked me to scrub in and see that the nurses passed the right instruments.

"What about your representative in New Jersey?" I asked.

"He's a nice guy," the surgeon said, "and he gets me what I need, but I know you do these cases, and I'd rather have you."

"Doctor," I said, "I'd love to be there."

On the day of surgery, as the surgeon started the case, I recognized immediately that he knew his craft. The way he moved, the comments he made, the assuredness with which he placed instruments in the hip cavity, bespoke his proficiency. Some surgeons, once inside, lose all sense of the anatomical positioning of different bones. They cannot find the body's landmarks. They "get lost in the wound," as their difficulty is termed. This doctor had no such problems. All he asked of me was to hold retractors and operate the acetabular cup positioner, which I was familiar with and he was not. The case went very well and took about two hours and twenty minutes, which is good time for a total hip. Several days later, the postman delivered a complete set of 1974 issues of the _Journal of Bone and Joint Surgery._ They were beautifully bound and accompanied by a note from the doctor thanking me for my time. I was deeply touched by his gift, not only because of the thought behind it but also because I read this journal regularly and had never bothered to have my own set bound.

Another surgeon sent me Volumes 1 and 2 of Campbell's _Operative Orthopedics,_ $150 worth of books. No note was attached, but I later learned from his secretary that he knew I read orthopedic texts and would probably appreciate the books. I had attended several of his procedures but had done little more than observe, check instruments, and help with the acetabular cup positioner. This doctor was fully capable of doing his own surgery.

In another example of good medicine, I know a general surgeon who does orthopedic surgery even though he was originally trained to operate on gall bladders and the like and received no formal training as an orthopedist. But in the hospital where he works, general surgeons have considerable experience installing a device known as the Austin-Moore hip. It is not a total hip, but a steel-ball-and-shaft device used when the femoral head is fractured and cannot be repaired by other means. Dr. Peter Danus, I will call him, is a master at installing Austin-Moore hips, despite his lack of proper credentials as an orthopedic surgeon. He can finish a procedure in forty minutes, skin to skin, which is extremely fast. Yet he never sacrifices technical perfection. I wanted to see Dr. Danus in action, so I called and asked if I could attend one of his cases. On the day of the procedure, I did not scrub, and was there as an observer only. I immediately noticed that once the patient was brought in and Dr. Danus finished scrubbing, the door to the operating room was closed. The nurses never left the room for extra instruments. Everything they needed was already in place on the scrub nurse's table.

The Austin-Moore procedure is not considered as glamorous as total hip implants in the surgical world. But it is a very exacting kind of surgery: the prosthesis must fit perfectly or the patient will suffer great pain. One unusual aspect is that after the initial incision is made, low on the patient's buttock, the surgeon manually dislocates the hip. The patient lies on his side with the injured hip up. The doctor flexes the thigh to a right angle and turns the angled leg inward until the patient's foot points directly toward the ceiling.

If the surgeon applies too much force, he can fracture the femur instead of dislocating it. There are other pitfalls. The neck of the femur must be cut in exactly the right plane or the prosthesis will not fit. The prosthesis is not attached with bone cement and the surgeon does not hollow the femoral shaft as he does in a total hip procedure, for this would result in a loose fit. Instead, he removes bone a bit at a time with special chisels and rasps.

All these steps Dr. Danus completed with such skill that watching him operate was a pleasure. When it came time to install the prosthesis, I knew it would fit. Dr. Danus checked to see if the head of the prosthesis fit into the acetabulum, which is largely a matter of feel. He then gently inserted the stem down the shaft of the femur, pushing it with his hands. He popped the steel femoral head into the acetabulum, checked the leg by moving it in all directions, and closed the incision. Very few deep sutures were needed to close the wound because the Austin-Moore procedure is not as bloody as other total hip surgery. When the case ended, I knew it was the most skilled surgery I had ever seen. Dr. Danus possesses that rare ability to make his hands do exactly as his brain decrees. The man was born to be a surgeon, and if ever a movie were made to teach how to install an Austin-Moore prosthesis, he should be leading man.

Another surgical wonder I have witnessed several times is hand surgery. This brand of orthopedics I seldom see because it does not require many implants. Once I watched a doctor dissect a tendon that was causing a hand to contract. He worked with tiny instruments in a very small operative field. After the violence of hip surgery, it was a pleasure to see a procedure so delicate. The tiniest slip of the scalpel would have compromised the case. He reminded me of a seasoned diamond cutter whose every cut has to be perfect lest he ruin the entire jewel.

Even inexperienced doctors performed surgical marvels. I was once privileged to observe a total hip case in a hospital in Nassau County in 1975. The OR supervisor called me because these two orthopedic residents had never done a Charnley total hip before. They had done Müller hips, which are similar, but many surgeons could not transfer the technique successfully. These two could. When the case began, they encountered some trouble setting up the initial incision retractor (the U-shaped gadget I had often seen surgeons place upside down), and I showed them how to position it. From then on, it was their case. They went skin to skin in less than two hours, with no complications. Like finely synchronized machines, they completed all the steps in the Charnley total hip procedure. I felt they needed me like a third eye, yet it was a pleasure to watch such surgical skill.

I later learned that they had stayed up several nights prior to the case reading every piece of literature Dr. John Charnley ever wrote about his procedure. They also watched a movie I had loaned them. They prepared so well that the 120-plus steps of the Charnley procedure were recorded in their minds, not on a sheet of paper. I knew that when these doctors finished their residencies, they would be fine surgeons. From all I have heard since, they are.

A surgeon who planned to implant a Townley total knee once asked me to see him after office hours. That turned out to be 11 P.M. No sooner had I arrived than he was called to an emergency. I followed him to the hospital and at midnight showed him movies of the total knee procedure. Despite the late hour, he studied the patient's X rays and a femur and tibia with the implant inserted. His desk was littered with articles he had been reading about the procedure. Because the Townley knee comes in about a dozen different sizes, he asked me to scrub so that I could hand him the proper-sized implant quickly. I was not needed for anything else. The doctor finished the procedure so quickly and skillfully that it seemed he had done 150 total knees. Yet it was his first.

Another surgeon, before doing a total ankle case, went to the morgue and practiced on a cadaver. He watched movies about the procedure. He read the literature. And, for good measure, he telephoned the Mayo Clinic doctor who invented the total ankle, just to be sure that he had done everything humanly possible for his patient.

I have known doctors who referred their patients rather than take on procedures they could not handle. In effect, they gave up income rather than risk a bad result for the patient. Such doctors prefer to tell a patient, "These total knees are still experimental, Mrs. Smith. Let's wait a few years until they're perfected." If the patient persists, that doctor will send her to a medical center where hundreds of total knee cases are handled.

Doctors have asked me, "Bill, you're always in the City. Who do you think is doing the best knee right now?"

I would answer, "It's this guy uptown," or "It's this guy midtown."

I have seen doctors telephone a colleague in New York City and refer the case. One surgeon in the Port Jefferson area of Long Island treated a woman with a severely arthritic knee about five years. Finally, he could suggest nothing except surgery to relieve her pain, but he did not feel qualified to implant a total knee prosthesis. I think his feeling was "I may not be the doctor who cures her, but I'm sure as hell not going to be the doctor who cripples her." So he referred her to another surgeon who implanted a total knee. Doctors like these—who give up $3000 fees rather than risk bad results for the patients—I respect.

But this is not how the entire orthopedic world operates. As a result, I performed surgery on the entire human skeleton: ankles, tibias, knees, femurs, hips, elbows, spines, skulls. I implanted medullary rods, Jewett nails, hip screws, bone plates, total knees, elbows, and hips. I even once pinned a fractured femur on a Great Dane. I have observed, but not participated in, abdominal surgery, oral surgery, and ear-nose-throat surgery. I have watched, in utter amazement, surgeons do a Caesarean section and lift a new human being from a mother's body. I have performed surgery in five states, including New York, but the number of times I have laid hands on patients I will never reveal, for the total would frighten the reader more than the context of this book intends.

FOURTEEN
UNMASKED

One day in the early fall of 1976, I received a telephone call from Neill Rosenfeld, an investigative reporter for *Newsday*. His name, like the others in this chapter, is real. He told me he had been looking into the Dr. Ashkenazy incident at Smithtown General Hospital. While doing so he had learned that I had been involved in a lot of surgery. I told him that I didn't want to talk to him.

A few weeks later he telephoned again. I did not return the call. After that, he started leaving phone messages daily. I realized I was dealing with a good, persistent reporter who knew he had a story, but as yet had no idea of its magnitude. Finally, I called and asked him to stop leaving messages because I had nothing to say to him.

I heard nothing further from Mr. Rosenfeld until midsummer 1977, when an operating-room nurse told me that he had visited her home asking about my surgical activities. At that point I went to some of the doctors involved to warn them that trouble might be brewing. I suggested to one that we decide how to handle the problem.

"Don't worry about Rosenfeld," he said. "We'll take care of it."

"Okay, if that's the way you want to handle it, fine."

One of my salesmen was making sales rounds with me that day, and when I left the doctor's office I told him, "I just tried to tip him off that the shit is going to hit the fan, and he didn't want to believe it. How can he be so complacent?"

"Sure, he's complacent," he said. "He's a doctor, and doctors are beyond reproach."

"Yeah," I said, "I forgot." And we went back to work selling orthopedic equipment.

Soon afterward, in August 1977, I received a phone call from Matthew L. Lifflander, Counsel and Director of the Medical Practice Task Force, Assembly of the State of New York. Earlier that January Stanley Steingut, Speaker for the New York State Assembly, had announced that two legislative committees would conduct a joint full-scale investigation of questionable medical practices in New York. It was heralded as the most comprehensive review of the regulation of the medical profession ever undertaken by an American legislative body, and was expected to continue two years. Matthew Lifflander, special counsel to Mr. Steingut, headed the probe of unnecessary hospitalization and unnecessary surgery, Medicaid fraud, rising malpractice insurance costs, physician's financial conflicts of interest, fragmentation of patient care, falsification of hospital records to conceal malpractice and, to quote the Speaker, the "conspiracy of silence" that protects errant physicians. The investigation was to include "ghost surgery," or instances "where parties contract with one physician to do surgery and wake up to find someone else did it." At the time, the public presumed that by "someone" Steingut meant another surgeon.

But the Task Force had learned otherwise, and Mr. Lifflander did not waste words when he telephoned me:

"We have received testimony that you've been doing surgery in a number of locations, and I'd appreciate it if you would come into my office to discuss the matter."

"Mr. Lifflander," I said, "I have no intention of seeing you now or at any time."

"Mr. MacKay, I really feel that you ought to come in here at your earliest convenience." His voice was patient, and kind, but I also know that he knew he had me cornered.

Thus I was subpoenaed to appear in Matthew Lifflander's

office on September 20, 1977. I brought my attorney, Leonard J. Meiselman, and we sat in a large conference room with Lifflander, a court stenographer from Albany, and New York State Assemblyman Alan G. Hevesi, Democrat from Queens and chairman of the Committee. I testified under oath for the next four hours, describing more than a dozen cases. Lifflander told me I might have to testify at public hearings his committee would hold within the month.

But, before Lifflander's public hearings ever took place, I was contacted by the Suffolk County District Attorney's Office by Mr. Albert Araneo of the Frauds Bureau. His message, in essence, was "Come see me in Hauppauge, or I'll send somebody after you." I went to his office one evening at five o'clock. As I sat there answering his questions, I was smiling a lot, and finally he said, "You think this is funny?"

"I think we should get something straight right away."

"What's that?" he said.

"When I'm laughing, I'm scared. If I don't laugh, I'm going to cry, and I'd rather laugh."

Then he brought in a police officer, Russ Crosley, who was assigned to the District Attorney's office as an investigator. Araneo produced a skeletal chart of the body, and asked me to explain what happened during the Mirando case, which is the case they were then investigating.

We talked for more than two hours, and as I was leaving at about seven-thirty, Officer Crosley insisted upon escorting me to my car.

"Why?" I asked.

"If anybody threatens you or your family, I want to know about it immediately."

Several days later, Araneo told me I would be subpoenaed to appear before a Suffolk County grand jury concerning the Mirando case. More than two years had passed since I hurried from the Harbor Hills golf course to repair his hip. Now, I learned, he claimed he suffered forty-nine separate injuries, from a two-inch difference in the length of his legs to a worsened spinal-disc problem. He said he spent most of his time in wheelchairs, one for upstairs, one for downstairs, and one for the car.

Only after Mirando had filed a $46-million malpractice suit against Lipton and Massoff and was called to testify before the Suffolk County Grand Jury did he learn of my role during his operation. His reaction, as *Newsday* recounted, was: "I hold no malice against the salesman. Without him, I probably wouldn't be alive." I felt gratified that Mirando credited me with saving his leg and perhaps his life. But I also felt saddened.

Now I would meet Mirando face to face. While I waited to testify in the Suffolk County Criminal Courts Building in Riverhead, Long Island, I was ushered into an office where I was sequestered from the other witnesses. I stepped out into the corridor for a cigarette just as Mirando's wife wheeled him off the elevator. As he passed me, I wanted desperately to speak to the man, but I feared what his reaction might be. So I remained silent.

When my turn came to testify before the grand jury, I was led into a room resembling an amphitheater. I sat against the wall, facing a microphone and about twenty-five people of all ages and types: old women in housedresses, young women in fancy suits, young men in business attire, middle-aged men in workmen's clothes. Far atop the sloping half-moon of chairs was a table with four or five gentlemen seated behind it. I never learned who they were.

The hearing was run by Al Araneo, who stood behind a docket to my left and asked questions: Did you touch Mr. Mirando? (Yes). Were you called off the golf course to perform surgery? (Yes). Did you put his femur back together? (Yes). Was Dr. Lipton there? (Yes). The grand jury confined itself to the Mirando case and I confined myself to the testimony I had given in Matthew Lifflander's office. I did not testify about any other cases.

As I was leaving the hearing room, I saw one of the doctors from Smithtown General walk in. "Hi, how are you?" he said. My spirits sank as I rode down the elevator. I had been assured that nobody would see me coming or going. Now the word would get out.

Three days after I testified before the grand jury, I was awakened from a deep sleep by a telephone call at eleven at night. A strange man's voice said, "MacKay, you can't watch your family and your children all the time. Stop talking to the authorities." And the phone clicked in my ear.

Then the press pounced. The various investigations had led to an article by Neill Rosenfeld in *Newsday* on October 28, 1977, telling the public for the first time that medical-equipment salesmen had operated in three Suffolk County hospitals. The next day *Newsday* ran a story about the Mirando case and the fact that a salesman (unnamed) had operated on him more than six hours. That was Saturday. The following Monday, October 31, *Newsday* informed the world that the salesman who had operated on Mirando was William MacKay.

Suddenly the telephone started ringing off the hook. Calls came from the major TV news networks, BBC, Canadian Broadcasting Company, the *National Enquirer, New York Post, The New York Times, Time,* and *Newsweek.*

Despite threats and entreaties, I gave interviews to no one but Neill Rosenfeld of *Newsday.* And this I did in an attempt to fend off other reporters and tell my side of the story. When Rosenfeld's story appeared on November first, it stimulated even more press interest. My wife answered the telephone every fifteen minutes during the day while I was at work. Reporters besieged my home. A newspaperman climbed over my fence and one night, while I was emptying the garbage, I was accosted by two reporters as I walked down the driveway.

The day after that story appeared, Suffolk County District Attorney Henry F. O'Brien held a press conference to announce that a grand jury had handed down three indictments after a six-week investigation growing out of information gathered by Lifflander's group.

The first indictment charged Dr. David Lipton, Dr. Harold Massoff, nurse Lorna Salzarullo, the anesthesiologist, and Smithtown General Hospital with second-degree assault in the Mirando case. The charge was brought under a law prohibiting the drugging of a person without his consent "for other than lawful medical or therapeutic treatment." Franklin Mirando, the indictment alleged, was anesthetized a second time without his consent so that I could illegally practice medicine. Nobody was charged with permitting the unlicensed practice of medicine—a misdemeanor—because the two-year statute of limitations for that offense had already expired.

A second indictment alleged that Lipton had falsified business records by omitting my name from the surgeon's report he had filed so that my participation in the operation would remain secret. A third indictment accused Lorna Salzarullo and Smithtown General Hospital of the same felony by omitting my name from the operating room log.

All were arraigned in the New York State Supreme Court in Riverhead, Long Island, on November 2, 1977. All pleaded innocent. All were released without bail. Lawyers for Smithtown General Hospital, however, declined to enter a plea of innocent or guilty, claiming that the hospital had been improperly charged. It had been indicted as if it were a corporation, not a partnership, they said, and there is no criminal liability for a partnership.

As the indictments were announced, a State Supreme Court Justice, at the request of the Suffolk County District Attorney's Office, signed an order empaneling a special grand jury to investigate other alleged instances of salesmen in surgery at Suffolk County hospitals.

Nassau County District Attorney Denis Dillon said his office would make inquiries to learn if similar happenings had occurred in his jurisdiction.

Matthew Lifflander met with district attorneys in Nassau County and Queens to give them information he had gathered and to avoid duplication of effort.

The Suffolk County District Attorney's Office sent information about the indictments to the county medical society and the American Medical Association for appropriate action.

Two days after the indictments were announced, the Joint Commission on Accreditation of Hospitals announced that it would investigate allegations that Smithtown General allowed salesmen in surgery.

From Washington, D.C., came word that the Department of Health, Education and Welfare had instructed the New York State Health Department, which inspects hospitals for Medicare eligibility, to determine whether allegations were true that I was allowed to perform surgery at Smithtown. The hospital faced possible loss of Medicare reimbursement, which could lead to loss of Blue Cross reimbursement, which in turn might force the hospital to close.

Speculation grew that the investigations would spread and, on November 3, 1977, *The New York Times* quoted Matthew Lifflander as saying "What we find here will have national implications."

Meanwhile, the medical community registered its reactions. The Nassau County Medical Society said it was "unaware of any ethical or improper practices" but would be happy to cooperate with investigations into such instances. The Suffolk County Medical Society deplored the "extreme publicity" surrounding the events of the previous week and predicted that they would cause "a serious undermining of confidence of people in their physicians and in their medical institutions."

The American College of Surgeons, American Hospital Association, and Joint Commission on Accreditation of Hospitals issued statements that they had never heard of any cases of salesmen actually participating in operations.

Officials of the American Academy of Orthopedic Surgeons were unavailable for comment.

A short time later, the Task Force heard testimony that salesmen for the United States Surgical Corporation of Stamford, Connecticut, had participated in more than 900 operations and had "scrubbed in" on more than 3000 operations in New York State during the past five years. The company is the sole manufacturer and marketer of Auto Suture surgical staplers in the U.S., devices that eliminate the need for time-consuming suturing with needle and thread. In one instance, it was alleged, a surgeon and salesman raced each other to see who could suture a patient's leg faster.

Meanwhile, on November 8, Patrick Henry, a Republican, defeated Democrat Henry O'Brien in his bid for a second term as District Attorney of Suffolk County. During the campaign, Henry charged that the indictments of the hospital and medical practitioners had been designed to enhance his opponent's bid for re-election.

Other events followed swiftly:

• New York State Assemblyman Alan Hevesi postponed public hearings by the Task Force until December in order to investigate "new information" that certain abuses might be more widespread than originally indicated.

• The attorney for Smithtown General Hospital asked Acting Supreme Court Justice Joseph Jaspan to dismiss charges against the hospital of second degree assault and falsifying business records. The attorney argued that a grand jury cannot indict a partnership. Judge Jaspan promised a decision within ten days.

• Judge Jaspan refused to dismiss charges against Smithtown General Hospital. (The Appellate Division of the New York State Supreme Court later overruled him.)

• Attorneys for the two surgeons, anesthesiologist, and nurse indicted in the Mirando case asked Judge Jaspan to dismiss the charges. Their motion argued that the State Assembly Medical Practice Task Force and Henry O'Brien had manipulated the news media for political advantage and had made a fair trial impossible. Judge Jaspan said he would decide in January whether to dismiss the charges.

Doctors, meanwhile, registered a wide range of reactions. Surgeons who once thanked me for joining them in the operating room now denied that I had ever been there. Other doctors called wanting to know whether I planned to implicate them. I felt sorry for them. Another doctor wanted to know what I had told the Suffolk County grand jury about a certain colleague of his. I reminded him that as a material witness I could not discuss my testimony with anybody even if I wanted to, which I did not.

Yet another doctor hand-wrote on his own prescription form that he would purchase no more soft goods—braces, slings, and the like—from the medical company I worked for as long as I was distributor, and that he would see to it that his hospital did likewise. Another doctor I had scrubbed with wrote to my company on hospital stationery and said if I was not fired he would transfer his business to another firm. Normally one letter would not carry much weight. But this doctor practices at one of the most prestigious medical institutions in New York, and is world-famous in his particular field. And a Brooklyn surgeon wrote stating he would no longer do business with a man whose testimony cost doctors their livelihoods and jeopardized their licenses.

Some doctors did, however, come to my defense. In an interview with Neill Rosenfeld, one surgeon acknowledged that some of his colleagues would not go into an operating room without me, and that my knowledge of implants was tremendous. In the midst of all the publicity, I was making sales calls one day in the Bronx and ran into a surgeon about to do a total hip case.

"How are you?" he asked.

"Fine, just making calls."

"I thought you'd be hiding out."

"I have nothing to hide," I said.

"Come on," he said, motioning toward the operating room. "We can talk in here."

So, in one of the most unusual invitations to surgery I have ever received, I scrubbed in on the case. I held retractors and helped him close the patient. It was a very straightforward, unspectacular total hip case. But here was a doctor who was unafraid of the publicity or other consequences that might come from having me there.

A short time later, on Christmas Eve, 1977, another surgeon

asked me to attend a medullary nailing case. One of my salesmen came into my den on the morning of December 23, while I was being interviewed by my collaborator for this book, and said that the OR supervisor at a hospital in Suffolk County had just called. A surgeon was having problems with a medullary nail and needed a special extracting instrument in a hurry because the nail was stuck. When he and I arrived at the hospital, we decided that the better part of valor demanded entry through the emergency room and up some back stairs. The operating-room supervisor met us and motioned toward one of the operating-room doors.

"They're having problems in there. They have a medullary nail jammed half in and half out of the femur, and they can't move it in either direction. Will you give them a hand?"

"Who is the surgeon?" I asked.

I paused to consider her answer. "Sure, I'll give him a hand."

The reason I hesitated is that, candidly, there were certain doctors I had no intention of getting involved with. I was in enough trouble. But this surgeon has talent and integrity, and I had scrubbed with him before. I put on greens and a mask, and entered the OR.

"Hi, Bill. Boy, I'm glad you're here. I've got a fifteen-millimeter nail jammed against cortical bone [the dense outer layer], and I'm afraid if I move it, I'll fracture the femur longitudinally. I already have a midshaft fracture."

"How far above the fracture line is the nail?" I asked. He told me. "Okay, I'll go scrub and give you a hand."

The assistant surgeon, upon hearing that I was about to become involved in the operation, immediately left the room, muttering something about office hours. The primary surgeon looked at me and said, "Fuck him. He's useless anyway. That's why I'm in this goddam jam!"

When I returned from the sinks, the surgeon asked if I had brought the extractor. "No, I didn't have one in the office. Do you have a pair of vise grips?" The scrub nurse handed them to me, and I tightened them on the upper end of the Kuntscher medullary nail, which had been driven through the greater trochanter and straight down the femoral canal, parallel to the bone. The mistake the surgeon had made was using a nail so large it would not hammer all the way down. I took a mallet and hit the vise grips from below. The nail would not budge.

"Doctor, you're going to have to make another incision

farther down the leg so we can manipulate this nail from the lower end."

"Are you sure, Bill?"

"I don't see where we have a choice," I replied.

He thought it over, then prepped the leg with Betadine and made a two-inch incision about seven inches below the greater trochanter. When retractors were in place, I pried the fracture open with a small osteotome until there was at least an inch of space between the two bone ends. They parted easily. I then drove an awl, which is pointed like an icepick, against the bottom of the nail.

"Hand me another mallet." The scrub nurse opened a new surgical pack and handed me one.

"Here is what we're going to do," I told the surgeon. "You hit your vise grips from beneath when I give the signal, and I will hit the awl at the same time. If the nail has pressure from two points, we might be able to move it."

"Okay," he said, "it's worth a try." I aimed my mallet.

"Ready? On the count of three, one-two-three, whack." Simultaneously, we struck and felt the nail move slightly.

"All right," I said. "Let's do it again, but first move your vise grips farther down toward the greater trochanter." My idea was that since the Kuntscher nail is clover-leaf-shaped with an open side, the vise grips might compress it and make it easier to move.

"Good idea," he said, and moved the vise grips.

"Ready? One-two-three, whack." And the nail slid out. A look of relief crossed the surgeon's face: "You know, this is really something. The last guy in the world who should be here today is Bill MacKay, with all the controversy surrounding you right now. But when I'm in trouble, you're the only guy I want."

When I left the hospital, I was proud that this doctor thought enough of my surgical skills to want me in his operating room. And I am grateful to him for having the courage to invite me.

A month later, on February 9, 1978, *The New York Times* reported that the new Suffolk County District Attorney, Patrick Henry, said the Mirando case indictments might be thrown out of court. "In my opinion there is a very serious question as to whether there is sufficient evidence" to sustain the indictments, he said. Then he went further, saying he was not sure he would carry the prosecution forward even if the indictments were upheld. The matter should be handled within the medical profession, not the courts. Mr. Henry added that related investigations had been suspended pending a ruling on the Mirando indictments.

The next day, Judge Jaspan dismissed criminal assault charges against Smithtown General Hospital, Lipton, Massoff, the anesthesiologist, and nurse Salzarullo. However, he refused to dismiss a felony charge against Lipton and Salzarullo for alleged criminal falsification of hospital records.

Jaspan ruled that the assault charges did not fit the criminal statutes cited in the preceding November's indictments. They had cited a section of the State Criminal Code prohibiting administration of a general anesthetic to a victim in order to commit a crime such as robbery. The anesthetic, Jaspan wrote in his opinion of February 10, 1978, was administered to help Franklin Mirando by implanting a total hip. "The conduct of the defendants, however ill-advised, was designed in good faith to achieve that result," the judge concluded. Thus the defendants did not act with the mental culpability required to commit assault.

But his decision regarding the assault charges, Judge Jaspan added, did not deal with the issue, as presented by the grand jury, that "Dr. Lipton abdicated his role as surgeon in that operating room and permitted the judgment and skills of a layman to prevail. Mr. MacKay's involvement in the surgical procedure extended far beyond instructions as to the use of manner of implant of a device he sold." Jaspan added: "The role of Dr. Harold Massoff is not so easily categorized, but in view of the finding herein need not be further explored."

At the time the judge refused to dismiss felony charges against Dr. David Lipton and nurse Lorna Salzarullo for alleged criminal falsification of hospital records to conceal my presence in the operating room because he found the evidence legally sufficient to support these indictments.

Meanwhile, the special grand jury empaneled in early November to investigate the extent of salesmen in surgery in Suffolk County hospitals was allowed to go quietly out of existence.

And what became of the public officials who had investigated the situation?

• Al Araneo, the assistant district attorney who brought the indictments against the doctors, nurse, and hospital in Suffolk County, was transferred to a minor post. He left the District Attorney's office and entered private law practice.

• Detective Russ Crosley, who had been assigned to the

Frauds Bureau in the District Attorney's office as investigator in the Mirando case and other matters, was transferred to a beat in Bayshore, Long Island.

• Detective Fred Kruger, another Frauds Bureau investigator who was present when I testified about the Mirando case, was demoted and transferred.

• Salvatore A. Alamia, chief prosecutor for the Frauds Bureau, was transferred to a job handling traffic misdemeanors.

As for me, the orthopedic device company I represented asked me to resign.

On June 19, 1978, Patrick Henry, the District Attorney of Suffolk County, filed an affidavit asking the dismissal of the indictment against David Lipton (see the complete affidavit and supporting documents in Appendix A). As this book went to press, I learned the dismissal had been granted.

The indictment charging Nurse Salzarullo with the crime of Falsifying Business Records in the First Degree was dismissed by Justice Joseph Jaspan on June 23, 1978, in response to a motion for dismissal filed by Patrick Henry, the District Attorney of Suffolk County. In support of the motion for dismissal (a complete copy is found in Appendix B), District Attorney Patrick Henry relied primarily on the inability to prove that Nurse Salzarullo had the primary responsibility for including MacKay's name in the hospital log for the Mirando operation.

FIFTEEN

POST-OP

A book such as this raises the question: What should come of it? It is not enough to merely expose abuses in which doctors use medical-equipment salesmen to supplement or supply knowledge doctors should have in the first place. Those abuses must end. I consider it deplorable that a minority of doctors allow ghost surgery to take place. By doing so they tarnish the reputations of their conscientious colleagues, who are in the majority.

Yet the surgeons who invited me into their operating rooms and allowed me to touch their patients never, I believe, meant to harm them. Their motive was to give those patients the best possible care available at that moment. I have never met a doctor who allowed anybody to do surgery unless he believed that person, *at that moment*, could do it better than he. No doctor can be well versed in every possible disaster that might arise. Sometimes, despite a surgeon's talent and technical expertise, the operation is not, and cannot be, a success. The mechanical nature of the specialty makes this particularly true of orthopedics.

Still, I feel that too many orthopedic surgeons I encountered failed to do their homework. Technology is no excuse. Modern total hip surgery has been around since the early 1960s, and even though artificial hips have changed frequently, along with the surgical technique for implanting them, every professional must keep abreast of his art, especially when it affects human life. If an airline mechanic fails to keep up with engine design and causes a plane crash through poor workmanship, would the victims and survivors forgive him? Or if an airline pilot was not checked out on a new type of plane he was to fly, can you imagine the congressional investigation that would be held when his plane crashed, killing hundreds of people?

If I were a surgeon, I would never allow another person to touch my patient. Yet I touched the patients of many surgeons. How do I reconcile my ideals and my actions? I was part of a sad state of affairs through necessity: the need to sell medical equipment and earn a living, plus the more vital need to keep somebody's arm or leg in one piece. Supposing I were to walk down the street tomorrow and see a man struck by an automobile. I would stop and assist him. Similarly, when I was in an operating room, I stepped in, not because I had practiced the procedure dozens of times but because those surgeons needed help and I was willing to give it. Franklin Mirando, for example, was a person in need, and I helped him.

Dr. Denton A. Cooley, the famous heart surgeon, once told *Medical World News* reporter Mark Bloom, who was writing about my role in the Mirando case, that orthopedics is "sort of a branch of carpentry. If somebody knows a better way to put a screw in, maybe he ought to demonstrate it." In that case, and many others, I believe I knew a better way.

Yet I must be careful about stating my limitations. I am, in Dr. Cooley's idiom, a bone carpenter, not a surgeon. Unlike an orthopedic surgeon who has a basic understanding of the entire human body, its functions and disorders, my expertise is confined to the skeleton itself. I do not claim to know anything about the circulatory or digestive systems, or even the nervous and muscular systems. My specialty is skeletal anatomy, particularly the repair of hips and knees.

All my life I could always make my hands do anything my mind told them. When I was young, I could hold the reins in a way that told a horse what I wanted. My hands tinkered inside automobile engines and banged auto bodies back into shape. In their finest moments, my hands held broken bones together inside a human body, picked cement fragments out of the narrowest of spaces, and sensed when a bone screw needed another turn. At my head's bidding, all this my hands could do. Still, I never was or could be a doctor. My training was self-training, my services were emergency services, my skills were limited.

Looking back, I can say that I enjoyed doing surgery. It was probably the greatest experience of my life. And I wish the medical profession had some place for an individual like myself who has special skills and experience of value to doctors. But there is no place for me. Hopefully, this book will help in the struggle to achieve legislation making ghost surgery illegal. No doctor should ever let a layman do surgery for him.

Efforts of the Medical Practice Task Force have led to legislation now pending in the New York State Assembly to prohibit surgical-supply salesmen and other unauthorized persons who are assisting a surgeon from touching a patient during surgery. This bill would also make any surgeon who permits such participation in surgery guilty of professional misconduct and a felony.

This legislation arose after the Task Force unearthed instances—aside from the ones I was involved in—of surgical-supply salesmen regularly scrubbing for surgery. One held a prosthetic knee device in place with his hands for an orthopedic surgeon. Another admitted to having used endoscopic instruments, which allow visual inspection of any cavity of the body. An ophthalmologist allowed "operating room technicians" he trained himself to handle and/or suture delicate portions of patients' eyes during surgery. And salesmen of automatic suturing devices in hundreds of instances were called upon to handle (and in some cases to actually operate) the devices while attached to human tissue during surgery.

The bill acknowledges the value of having experts present in the operating room to answer questions. And it requires that the surgeon and operating-room supervisor record in the operating room log the name and purpose of anybody present. But in no case will unauthorized persons be allowed to touch a patient.

A second proposal, which grew out of Task Force investigations, would prohibit ghost surgery and require that patients know the identity of all surgeons who perform, supervise, or participate in their surgery. The Task Force estimated that from fifty to eighty-five percent of the surgery in teaching hospitals is ghost surgery—performed by residents without the knowledge of the patients. The bill also requires that, except in an emergency, the surgeon the patient chooses perform and directly supervise the operation. This bill passed the Assembly, but at this writing, was stalled in the Senate.

Still another proposal—The Quality of Health Care Act of 1978—would subject a physician who performs unnecessary surgery to the loss of his license to practice. This legislation would create a board to establish and enforce health-care standards and a single authority, the Office of Health Systems Management, to coordinate a variety of new medical and hospital monitoring programs and some already in existence. The office would develop ways to assess the quality of health care, control hospital costs, and allow patients to recover payments for unnecessary, incompetent, or substandard care. It would publicize the performance records of hospitals to help the public and physicians choose the best possible hospitals and avoid the worst. Further, the bill would require that physicians receive continuing education as a condition for renewal, every two years, of their medical licenses. At present these licenses are granted for life.

I support such legislation, for if salesmen are prohibited by law from touching a patient, and problem physicians are identified and disciplined, surgeons will be forced to do their homework. If surgeons do more homework (being intelligent individuals, or they would not be doctors in the first place) they will do better surgery, which is what everybody wants.

Other, equally important, legislation initiated by the Task Force and already made law requires hospitals and all health-care professionals to report any instances of misconduct or impairment of physicians. Any doctor failing to report an errant colleague could lose his license to practice. The proposals would also grant immunity from prosecution to anybody who, in good faith, reports medical misconduct. A study of more than a thousand complaints filed with the State Health Department during a recent sixteen-month period demonstrates the need for such immunity. Of the thousand complaints against physicians, thirty-one came from doctors, thirty-seven from medical societies, four from nurses, and three from the insurance industry. The rest came from patients, who are probably the least aware of what they have to complain about.

Doctors, obviously, do not police themselves. This leaves only the American public to take physicians to task. Yet we are doing a terrible job of monitoring the medical care we receive.

We tolerate the sketchy descriptions of our ailments, the vague advice on treatment. The average patient says, "Doctor, I have a pain in my hip."

The doctor says, "Let me look at it."

He looks. "You have a problem here, Mr. Jones. We're going to have to do an operation."

And the patient unquestioningly accepts the doctor's verdict.

Another patient says, "Doctor, my knee's getting worse. I know it's arthritic."

The doctor takes some X rays. "You're right, Mrs. Smith. You have an arthritic knee. We're going to give you an implant."

The times, thank God, are changing. As recently as five years ago, if a patient had demanded to see his chart in a hospital or asked a nurse, "What's my blood pressure," she would have smiled and answered, "You're fine" or "Ask your doctor."

Today, some states have laws saying that patients can have access to their records. Yet millions of Americans, who grew up in the age of the nonanswer, do not even bother to ask. That generation will eventually be replaced by a more demanding, medically informed breed of patient. And then blind trust in the surgeon will cease.

Such happenings are in the future. The problem for the contemporary consumer of medical services is to find a _good_ surgeon. Selecting a good surgeon is tricky, for the choice is usually made upon the referral of another physician at a time of maximum stress. My experiences, especially with competent surgeons I have known, suggest some ways to make the best choice.

First, ask about the procedure: Why do I need it? What are the alternatives? What does the surgery entail? How long will I be hospitalized? How long will recovery take? What will it cost? Do you foresee any problems with my case? What are the chances of success?

Second, observe how the doctor responds. Does he answer questions fully? Is he vague? Is he impatient? Does he oversimplify, refuse to answer, or plead "You wouldn't understand"? In general, the more secretive he is, the more he may have to hide. The doctor who takes time to explain every step of a procedure is a confident, and probably competent, surgeon.

Third, beware of wild, outrageous promises, such as "You'll be walking in two weeks after your total hip operation." A responsible doctor will tell that same patient "You'll be able to walk much better than before, you'll be free of pain, but it will be months before you can live a normal life again."

Fourth, check out the doctor. Ask him directly: How many total hips (or whatever) have you done? How successful have they been? How well-equipped is the hospital, and how familiar is the staff with the procedure? Then ask the doctor for names of other patients who have had the procedure he recommends. Telephone them and ask about the problems and benefits they have experienced. A secure surgeon should be willing to provide this information. In fact, the doctor who implanted a total knee in my mother *offered* to let her speak to other patients he had treated. This kind of cross-examination may come as a shock to many doctors, but it is their responsibility to answer, and the patient's responsibility to ask, because we get the kind of medical care we deserve.

As for my own future, this book ends my surgical enterprises, as well as my career as a medical-equipment salesman. And, having no more to say, Bill MacKay, the salesman/surgeon, herewith turns in his gloves. I loved doing surgery, I miss doing surgery, and I would like to do surgery if asked.

But I also feel—and this book explains why—I should never be asked again.

APPENDIX A

SUPREME COURT OF THE STATE OF NEW YORK
COUNTY OF SUFFOLK

---------------------------- X

THE PEOPLE OF THE STATE
OF NEW YORK   :   NOTICE OF
                                                  MOTION

    -against-   :
                                                  Indictment
DAVID LIPTON,   :   Number
                                                  2051-77
      Defendant.   :

---------------------------- X

SIRS:

    PLEASE TAKE NOTICE, that upon the annexed affidavit of the HONORABLE PATRICK HENRY, District Attorney of Suffolk County, sworn to on the 19th day of June, 1978, and all other papers and proceedings heretofor had, the People of the State of New York will move this Court in Criminal Term Part II sitting in the H. Lee Dennison Building, Hauppauge, New York, on the 19th day of June, 1978, at

9:30 o'clock in the forenoon or as soon thereafter as counsel can be heard for an order dismissing the indictment as against the defendant DAVID LIPTON in furtherance of justice pursuant to Criminal Procedure Law section 210.40.

Dated: Hauppauge, New York
June 19, 1978

Yours, etc.

PATRICK HENRY, ESQ.
District Attorney of Suffolk County
H. Lee Dennison Building
Veterans Memorial Highway
Hauppauge, New York 11787
(516) 979-2400

TO: ANGELO COMETA, ESQ.
Attorney for Defendant
40 West 57th Street
New York, New York 10019

At a Term of the Supreme Court, held in
and for the County of Suffolk, at the
Courthouse thereof, H. Lee Dennison
Building, Veterans Memorial Highway,
Hauppauge, New York, on the   day of
June, 1978.

PRESENT:

HONORABLE JOSEPH JASPAN
Justice of the Supreme Court

-------------------------- X

THE PEOPLE OF THE STATE OF
NEW YORK   :
                                                         ORDER
    -against-   :   Indictment
                                                         Number
DAVID LIPTON,   :   2051-77

       Defendant.   :

-------------------------- X

    The People of the State of New York, by PATRICK
HENRY, District Attorney of the County of Suffolk, having
moved this Court by Notice of Motion dated June 19, 1978, for
an order dismissing indictment number 2051-77 and the said
motion having regularly come before this Court on June 19,
1978, and the matter having been submitted in behalf of the
moving party in support thereof, and the defendant having
made no opposition to the dismissal of the indictment,

    AND, on reading and filing the said Notice of Motion, the
affidavit of PATRICK HENRY, District Attorney of the County of Suffolk in support thereof, sworn to on June 19, 1978 and
upon the exhibit annexed thereto, and upon the affidavit
of   dated June   , 1978, submitted in reply to
the People's motion papers, and upon all of the proceedings
had herein and due deliberation having been had thereon,   ,

NOW, on motion of PATRICK HENRY, District Attorney of the County of Suffolk, it is

ORDERED, that indictment number 2051-77 charging the defendant DAVID LIPTON with the crime of Falsifying Business Records in the First Degree be and the same is hereby dismissed in furtherance of justice pursuant to section 210.40 of the Criminal Procedure Law.

ENTER,

_____

Justice of the Supreme Court

SUPREME COURT OF THE COUNTY OF SUFFOLK
STATE OF NEW YORK

-------------------------- X

THE PEOPLE OF THE STATE OF
NEW YORK   :
                                                      AFFIDAVIT
    -against-   :   Indictment
                                                      Number
DAVID LIPTON,   :   2051-77

      Defendant.   :

-------------------------- X

STATE OF NEW YORK)
) SS.:
COUNTY OF SUFFOLK)

    PATRICK HENRY, being duly sworn, hereby deposes
and says:
    1. I am the duly elected District Attorney of Suffolk
County, having assumed office on January 1, 1978.
    2. This affidavit is made upon information and belief in
support of a motion to dismiss indictment number 2051-77
against the defendant DAVID LIPTON, in furtherance of
justice, pursuant to Criminal Procedure Law section 210.40.
    3. On October 25, 1977, a Suffolk Grand Jury heard
evidence which resulted in an indictment for the crime of
Falsifying Business Records in the First Degree, a class E
felony, contrary to Penal Law section 170.10. DAVID LIP-
TON stands indicted by himself under number 2051-77;
however, indictment number 2052-77 was simultaneously
voted and handed up to the County Court of Suffolk County,
charging defendant DAVID LIPTON and four co-defendants
with the crime of Assault in the Second Degree, a class D
felony, in violation of Penal Law section 120.05(5). On November 2, 1977, the defendant appeared before the HONOR-
ABLE FRANK L. GATES, County Judge, for arraignment. A
plea of not guilty was entered by the defendant as to both
indictment numbers 2051-77 and 2052-77, and upon the
referral by the HONORABLE FRANK L. GATES of these

indictments to the HONORABLE JOSEPH JASPAN, Acting Justice of the Supreme Court, an order was thereafter made and entered affecting the removal of jurisdiction from the County Court to the Supreme Court, Suffolk County.

4. Thereafter, on February 10, 1978, this Court ordered that indictment number 2052-77 be dismissed as against all defendants therein. The same February 10, 1978, memorandum decision denied the defendant LIPTON'S motion to dismiss indictment number 2051-77 for reasons set forth at length therein.

5. A thorough and time-consuming review of all aspects of the prosecution's case against the defendant herein as well as all related cases involving the various other defendants in related indictments has been carried out by your deponent in collaboration with several members of my staff. The conclusions set forth below which are urged upon the Court as supporting grounds for dismissal of indictment number 2051-77 are the results of careful and detailed analysis conducted by the Office of the District Attorney.

6. There is abundant and persuasive evidence available to the prosecution, much of which was presented to the Grand Jury on October 25, 1977, that this defendant engaged in conduct constituting the crime of Unlawful Medical Practice, a misdemeanor pursuant to section 65.12 of the Education Law. Defendant LIPTON is an orthopedic surgeon, and in that capacity on July 3, 1975, performed hip surgery known as a total hip Arthroplasty upon patient FRANKLIN MIRANDO at Smithtown General Hospital. The defendant's criminal liability derived under Penal Law section 20.00, in that he solicited, requested, importuned and intentionally aided WILLIAM MACKAY, a salesman for the manufacturer of the surgical implant prosthesis utilized in the MIRANDO surgery, to carry out extensive and complex surgical procedures upon MIRANDO that the defendant himself was apparently incapable of successfully completing. Prosecution for the misdemeanor for which the defendant would have been accessorially liable was barred beyond July 3, 1977 (Criminal Procedure Law section 30.10(2-c)) by lapse of the two-year period of limitations. The Office of the District Attorney became aware of the events underlying these several cases in September, 1977, upon referral of the investigation from the New York State Assembly's Medical Practices Task Force. There being no circumstances present which would have affected exten-

sion of the period of limitations for the commencement of criminal action for the aforesaid misdemeanor, such prosecution was thereby barred when the investigation by this office began in September, 1977.

7. The indictment herein charges that the defendant LIPTON between July 3, 1975, and August 26, 1975, with intent to defraud and to conceal the crimes of Unauthorized Practice of Medicine and Assault omitted to make a true entry in his Operative Report, known also as the Surgeon's Report, in that he did not refer to participation of WILLIAM MAC-KAY, a person not authorized to practice medicine. By reason of the dismissal of indictment number 2052-77 and the reasons expressed therefor in the aforementioned February 10, 1978, memorandum decision, it has become the law of the case that the alleged crime of Assault was not committed. Therefore the only crime that could have allegedly been intended concealed was the Unauthorized Practice of Medicine. Any intent by defendant LIPTON to conceal in his Surgeon's Report the extensive nature of the comminuted femoral fracture caused by him during the July 3rd surgery on MIRANDO can, of course, not serve as a predicate for the aggravating element of the specific intent to conceal, as such conduct, while it may have constituted professional ineptitude or malpractice, was not of a criminal nature.

8. The indictment herein alleges a crime relatively distant in its gravamen from the acts of defendant LIPTON where true culpability lies, that is, his accessorial liability for the misdemeanor of Unauthorized Medical Practice, as discussed above. That prosecution therefor is barred by the lapse of the period of limitations is not a factor which should, in your deponent's opinion, provide justification for the derivative offense contained in the indictment herein which for reasons next discussed is untenable from the evidence which is known to the prosecution.

9. The alleged falsified document is an Operative Report. There appears to be no reason to style it a Surgeon's Report, as the indictment mentions. As an operative report the purpose or character of it is more easily defined as related to the details of the operation itself, and is compatible with the passive voice the defendant, its author, employs throughout the narrative to describe the surgical procedure. This factor would seem to make less necessary inclusion of the names of persons who carried out the steps and procedures. Stated

another way, the operation itself and not the person or persons who did it is the focus of the Operative Report in issue. Therefore, the exclusion of MACKAY'S name in the document is not inappropriate from a reading of the report on its face.

10. The Operative Report's only category which might arguably have called for inclusion of MACKAY'S name is "Assistant." This term is singular and lends itself to being interpreted as calling for the designated physician assistant. Nothing about this category suggests that others who assisted in some fashion should be included. It appears clear that various medical personnel usually assist in some way in every surgery. To read the term "Assistant" as meaning only those who physically contact the patient or manipulate surgical instruments is no more apparent than an interpretation that limits the "Assistant" to the physician who is designated to assist in the surgery. It appears that it has long been accepted practice for there to always be such a designated assisting surgeon for the purpose, among others, to complete the surgery in the event the primary surgeon can't continue for some reason. The designation of one such assistant surgeon is not incompatible with other physicians or technicians assisting in some fashion or to some extent. It is therefore equally reasonable to interpret the category of "Assistant" as calling for the surgeon designated in accordance with long accepted practice. Here, this assistant was defendant's partner, HAROLD MASSOFF, M.D., and this name is set forth, singularly, in the Operative Report in issue. It is noted also that nowhere on the document is there any provision for identifying persons who assisted as technicians, for example, the X-ray technicians or the anesthesiologist. Exclusion of any such provision for naming such persons who obviously provide needed assistance in the operation is supportive of an argument that this document is not intended to be exhaustive as to all persons who "assisted" in one way or another. DR. AARON CHAVES of the Department of Health Services of Suffolk County testified about such non-physician persons in the operating room. (pp. 133–137)

11. The discussion in the paragraph preceding goes to whether there was any duty imposed upon defendant LIPTON to include MACKAY'S name by the nature of his position. Although it may certainly be argued that the defendant's position as surgeon imposed upon him a duty to include

the appropriate or necessary information in the report, it seems clear that if the document itself did not require inclusion of MACKAY'S name, nothing in the nature of LIPTON'S position imposed such a duty. In summary, it is the position of the People that reasonable doubt exists that there existed such a duty.

12.   There is clearly no duty imposed by law which would have required the defendant to list MACKAY'S name as assistant. Pursuant to Public Health Law section 2803 in 1975 code provisions were established governing organization and administration of a hospital, and are set forth in 10 N.Y.C.R.R., Part 720. There is no provision therein which specifies what matters must be included in a doctor's "medical report," beyond a requirement that his report must be authenticated and signed in a timely fashion. Section 720.20(c), in referring to an "accurate and complete medical record," cannot be read as imposing a duty upon the defendant by law to have included MACKAY'S name in the document in issue. Section 720.13(G) requires a *hospital* to maintain a register of operations in a "bound book in the operating room suite." This must include, among other things, a list of the "surgeon, anesthetists, *assistants* and nurses" (emphasis supplied). Clearly this section is not applicable to the surgeon and imposed no particular duty upon the defendant as to his operative report, a document entirely distinct from the register of operations, addressed by section 720.13(g). However, the fact that there was another record which was required to contain names of "assistants," to wit, the operating room log at Smithtown General Hospital, and that this was evidently known to the defendant as chief of orthopedic surgery, lends support to an argument that he may not have perceived a duty to record all such names on his operative report. In the absence of a duty imposed by law upon the defendant to have included MACKAY'S name in the report and with reasonable doubt enshrouding the issue of a duty imposed by the nature of his position, there is then a failure of proof as to a necessary element of the offense of Falsifying Business Records in the First Degree.

13.   The reasons discussed in the preceding paragraphs pertaining to the issue of a duty to have reported MACKAY as an assistant appear to apply with comparable emphasis to the more troublesome element of the defendant's *mens rea:* the intent to defraud, which must include an intent to conceal

the commission of another crime. For if one concludes that the defendant had no duty to have included his identity on the Operative Report, logic dictates that no inference may flow as to the specific intent to defraud by reason of the omission of the MACKAY references. In that portion of this Court's memorandum decision of February 10, 1978, which discuss the sufficiency of the Grand Jury proof on the element of specific intent in this indictment the Court recognizes the inference of an intent to conceal the crime of Unlawful Medical Practice from the results produced. Premised upon inspection of the Grand Jury proof which views the evidence uncontradicted and unexplained, as, of course, the Court must upon such a motion to inspect and dismiss, such an inference of intent is possible where there has been a threshold finding of the existence of a duty upon the defendant, as discussed supra. However, the prosecution considers, following detailed assessment of its evidence, that there is no articulable proof that omission of the MACKAY reference in the defendant's Operative Report was, firstly, with the intent to defraud, and, secondly, that the intent to defraud included a design to conceal the crime of Unlawful Medical Practice. Although as discussed above it is the prosecution's contention that the defendant did commit this offense, without a finding of a duty or even that it was appropriate to have identified MACKAY in the Operative Report, there is missing the necessary logical nexus between the commission of that crime and a specific intent to conceal it by defendant's omission of the MACKAY reference.

14. Your deponent believes it to be particularly appropriate to combine the bringing of the within motion and another motion made simultaneously seeking dismissal of indictment number 2050-77 as against operating room supervisor LORNA SALZARULLO, with recommendations to the HONORABLE HUGH CAREY, Governor of the State of New York, that he sign without delay a bill expected to be sent to him from the state legislature before it recesses by the end of this week, the week of June 18th. As of the date this affidavit is made the bill has been passed overwhelmingly by the Assembly and its passage by the Senate is anticipated within the next three days. This legislation was generated and grew out of the same series of hearings conducted by the State Assembly's Medical Practices Task Force, led by Assemblyman ALAN G. HEVESI, Chairman of the Assembly Health

Committee, which referred evidence to this Office in September of 1977 leading to the investigation and eventual return of indictments as aforesaid. The bill would make it a felony for "surgical supply salesmen and other unauthorized persons" to "touch the human tissue of a patient during surgery." Further, under the proposed law a surgeon "who permits any unauthorized person to touch a patient" would also be guilty of a felony.

15. With dismissal of the indictments against defendants DAVID LIPTON and LORNA SALZARULLO, the prosecutions in Suffolk County of the various defendants under three related indictments will be brought to a close. Yet the investigation which resulted in these prosecutions has brought to light the grievous abuses in the operating room by certain members of the medical profession, and the occasional tragic harm to the unwary and trusting patient. It is from the insight afforded by this office's investigation and the need for more effective protection of the patient's interests that has become evident through it that your deponent believes it necessary and appropriate to make known to the governor the urgent recommendation of the Office of the District Attorney of Suffolk County that this bill be signed into law.

16. No previous application has been made for the relief sought herein.

17. Under all of the foregoing circumstances it would therefore be highly improbable that the People's proof upon trial would survive judicial scrutiny upon a motion made for a trial order of dismissal and most certainly would not be sufficient to establish the guilt of this defendant beyond a reasonable doubt. Accordingly, the People respectfully move this Court for a dismissal of indictment number 2051-77 as to defendant DAVID LIPTON in furtherance of justice pursuant to Criminal Procedure Law section 210.40.

PATRICK HENRY
District Attorney of Suffolk County

Sworn to before me this
19th day of June, 1978.

OPERATIVE REPORT

MIRANDO, FRANKLIN
#154237

DATE:	July 3, 1975
PREOPERATIVE DIAGNOSIS:	OSTEOARTHRITIS, RIGHT HIP
POSTOPERATIVE DIAGNOSIS:	SAME.
OPERATION:	TOTAL HIP AR-THROPLASTY, RIGHT.
SURGEON:	DAVID LIPTON, M.D.
ANESTHESIA:	GENERAL.
ASSISTANT:	HAROLD MASS-OFF, M.D.

PROCEDURE: The procedure was performed as described by Charnley with the prescribed prepped and draped extending from the base of the toes to the rib cage and draped appropriately. A long lateral incision was made extending from some 5 to 6 inches proximal to the greater trochanter and 5 to 6 inches distal along the lateral aspect of the hip, carried down to subcutaneous tissue. Appropriate muscles were divided and held retracted with the Charnley retractors. The greater trochanter was osteotomized and it and its attached musculature retracted superiorly. The joint capsule was opened and the neck of the femur osteotomized and the head delivered from the acetabulum. With the appropriate reamers the acetabulum was reamed and appropriate counter sinking holes were made to hold the cement. The central hole made by the centering drill was capped by a Mexican hat. The acetabulum was thoroughly irrigated, dried, Methacrylate was inserted and the Polyethylene cup inserted with the holder designed for this purpose and permitted to set. The excess Methacrylate was then trimmed away from around the cup so that there was no excess present. The cup holder was then removed and with aid of Rongeur the hardened Methacrylate was removed.

The intramedullary canal of the femur was then reamed with an additional portion of the neck removed as required to accept the stem prosthesis. A drill hole was fashioned in the proximal femur through which a wire was inserted to be utilized to secure the greater trochanter. The prosthesis was inserted and the test reduction was made and found to be satisfactory.

Intramedullary canal was cleared of all blood as best as could be done, was well irrigated and Methacrylate was inserted and the prosthesis inserted and held. When this was done patient was given intravenous Keflin.

EXHIBIT A

OPERATIVE REPORT   PAGE TWO

MIRANDO, FRANKLIN
#154237

After the prosthesis was set again an attempt at reduction was made. This time it was felt that the prosthesis had been inserted with too much anteversion resulting in repeated dislocation when the leg was held in neutral. It was felt that, at this time, the stem prosthesis should be removed and reinserted with less anteversion to prevent postoperative dislocation. While attempting to remove the prosthesis a crack in the proximal femur was developed. The prosthesis, however, was freed of the Methacrylate and this cement was then removed from the intramedullary canal so that the prosthesis could be then reinserted. Methylmethacrylate was then reinserted into the intramedullary canal, prosthesis again inserted with less anteversion. The fine crack in the proximal femur was secured with a 2 palm [sic] bands. The greater trochanter was secured with the heavy-duty wire after the hip was reduced and felt to be stable.

Throughout the procedure the wound was repeatedly irrigated with antibiotic solutions. The suction tubings were inserted and placed the suction as the wound was closed using interrupted 2-0 chromic catgut sutures for the deep fascia, interrupted 3-0 plain catgut suture for the subcutaneous tissue, interrupted 3-0 silk suture for the skin. Dry sterile dressing was applied. A hip abduction bolster was inserted between the patient's leg and he left the Operating Room in good condition.

DAVID LIPTON, M.D.
lb
D-8-26-75
T-8-26-75

APPENDIX B

SUPREME COURT OF THE STATE OF NEW YORK
COUNTY OF SUFFOLK

------------------------------- X

THE PEOPLE OF THE STATE OF
NEW YORK   :

    -against-   :

LORNA SALZARULLO,   :

       Defendant.   :

------------------------------- X

Indictment
Number
2050-77

NOTICE OF

SIRS:

    PLEASE TAKE NOTICE, that upon the annexed affidavit of the HONORABLE PATRICK HENRY, District Attorney of Suffolk County, sworn to on the 19th day of June, 1978, and upon the exhibits thereto annexed, and upon the indictment and all other papers and proceedings heretofor had, the People of the State of New York will move this Court in Criminal Term Part II sitting in the H. Lee Dennison Building, Hauppauge, New York, on the 19th day of June, 1978, at 9:30 o'clock in the forenoon or as soon thereafter as counsel can be heard for an order dismissing the indictment as against the defendant LORNA SALZARULLO in furtherance of justice pursuant to Criminal Procedure Law section 210.40.

Dated: Hauppauge, New York
        June 19, 1978

                Yours, etc.

                PATRICK HENRY, ESQ.
                District Attorney of Suffolk County
                H. Lee Dennison Building
                Veterans Memorial Highway
                Hauppauge, New York 11787
                (516) 979-2400

TO: LAWRENCE S. GOLDMAN
      Attorney for Defendant
      60 East 42nd Street
      New York, New York

At a Term of the Supreme Court, held in and for the County of Suffolk, at the Courthouse thereof, H. Lee Dennison Building, Veterans Memorial Highway, Hauppauge, New York, on the 23 day of June, 1978.

PRESENT:

HONORABLE JOSEPH JASPAN

Justice of the Supreme Court

-------------------------- X

THE PEOPLE OF THE STATE OF
NEW YORK

                          :

    -against-   :   ORDER
                                  Indictment
LORNA SALZARULLO,   :·   Number
                                  2050-77

      Defendant.   :

-------------------------- X

The People of the State of New York, by PATRICK HENRY, District Attorney of the County of Suffolk, having moved this court by Notice of Motion dated June 19, 1978, for an order dismissing indictment number 2050-77 and the said motion having regularly come before this Court on June 19, 1978, and the matter having been submitted in behalf of the moving party in support thereof, and the defendant having made no opposition to the dismissal of the indictment,

AND, on reading and filing the said Notice of Motion, the affidavit of PATRICK HENRY, District Attorney of the County of Suffolk in support thereof, sworn to on June 19, 1978, and upon the exhibits annexed thereto, and upon all of the proceedings had herein and due deliberation having been had thereon,

NOW, on motion of PATRICK HENRY, District Attorney of the County of Suffolk, it is

ORDERED that indictment number 2050-77 charging the defendant LORNA SALZARULLO with the crime of Falsifying Business Records in the First Degree be and the same is hereby dismissed in furtherance of justice pursuant to section 210.40 of the Criminal Procedure Law.

ENTER,

_____

Justice of the Supreme Court

SUPREME COURT OF THE COUNTY OF SUFFOLK
STATE OF NEW YORK

------------------------- X

THE PEOPLE OF THE STATE OF
NEW YORK

                        :

  -against-   :   AFFIDAVIT

LORNA SALZARULLO,   :   Indictment
                              Number
    Defendant.   :   2050-77

------------------------- X

STATE OF NEW YORK)
) SS.:
COUNTY OF SUFFOLK)

    PATRICK HENRY, being duly sworn, hereby deposes and says:

    1. I am the duly elected District Attorney of Suffolk County, having assumed office on January 1, 1978.

    2. This affidavit is made upon information and belief in support of a motion to dismiss indictment number 2050-77 as to the defendant LORNA SALZARULLO, in furtherance of justice, pursuant to Criminal Procedure Law section 210.40.

    3. On October 25, 1977, a Suffolk Grand Jury heard evidence which resulted in an indictment for the crime of Falsifying Business Records in the First Degree, a Class E felony, contrary to Penal Law section 175.10. Defendant SALZARULLO was jointly indicted with "Smithtown General Hospital" in a single pleading, and on November 2, 1977, the defendant herein appeared before the HONORABLE FRANK L. GATES, County Judge for arraignment. A plea of not guilty was entered by the defendant as to the within indictment, as well as to indictment number 2052-77, a companion indictment wherein defendant SALZARULLO stood accused along with four other defendants.

    4. Thereafter, on February 10, 1978, this Court ordered

that indictment number 2052-77 be dismissed as against all defendants. With respect to "Smithtown General Hospital" as a co-defendant on indictment number 2050-77, on March 10, 1978, an Order was made by the Appellate Division of the Supreme Court, Second Judicial Department, granting that defendant's application brought pursuant to Article 78 of the C.P.L.R., and prohibited the *nisi prius* court and the District Attorney of Suffolk County from further prosecution.

5.   In the aforementioned February 10, 1978, decision of this Court, the motion to dismiss the within indictment as against defendant SALZARULLO was denied for reasons set forth at length therein.

6.   A thorough and time-consuming review of all aspects of the prosecution's case against the defendant herein, as well as all related cases involving the several other defendants, has been carried out by your deponent in collaboration with several members of my staff. The conclusions set forth below which are urged upon the Court as supporting grounds for dismissal are the result of careful and detailed analysis conducted by the Office of the District Attorney.

7.   The indictment herein essentially accuses the defendant, in her capacity as the hospital's operating room supervisor, of failing to make a true entry in the operating room log, known also as the operating room register, by omitting the name of one WILLIAM MACKAY as an "assistant" in the July 3, 1975, hip operation performed on FRANKLIN MIRANDO.

8.   An indispensable element of the crime charged herein is proof that the omission of MACKAY'S name in the log was in violation of a duty imposed by law *or* by the nature of the defendant's position. It is clear that no duty is imposed by law which would have required the defendant to include MACKAY'S name. The New York Code of Rules and Regulations pertaining to a broad spectrum of hospital procedures addresses the necessity for maintaining an operating room log in section 720.13(G). But this section requires only that such a document be kept and that it contain six categories of information, but is silent as to who is responsible for keeping the register of operations. No "duty imposed by law" can be imputed to the defendant as operating room supervisor by reason of section 720.13(G).

9.   It was not in the nature of the defendant's position that she have primary responsibility for entries in the log or

register. The duty to make the appropriate and correct entries fell to a particular hospital employee, the operating room secretary. Although the Chief of Surgery testified before the Grand Jury that it was the defendant's responsibility as supervisor to maintain the operating room log, there is clear proof to the contrary. All entries made on the log of July 3, 1975, were made by the secretary and not the defendant. As a result of process served upon the hospital's administrator, this office is in possession of documents purporting to set forth particularized job descriptions for various employees of Smithtown General Hospital, including the positions of operating room supervisor and operating room secretary. Annexed hereto are true copies of these job descriptions, marked Exhibits A and B, reference to which demonstrates that the secretary "records operations in the Operating Room log book in legible manner," and the operating room supervisor "assumes responsibility for overall supervision of all cases booked in the Operating Room. . . ." The secretary was clearly supervised by the defendant but the defendant's job description excludes any reference to responsibility for the log. The conclusion appears inevitable, then, that in addition to there having been no duty imposed upon her by law, neither was there a duty imposed upon the defendant by the nature of her particular position to record MACKAY'S name as an assistant in the MIRANDO surgery.

10. Even if one were to advance a theory that the defendant's supervisory position imputed to her such a duty, logic would then preclude us from imputing a criminal intent to defraud to defendant SALZARULLO from the failure of her subordinate to record MACKAY'S name in the log. Of necessity additional affirmative proof would be needed that 1) the defendant herself knew MACKAY had "assisted" in the MIRANDO operation and 2) the defendant had actual knowledge that her subordinate, the operating room secretary, had omitted MACKAY'S name. Such proof is not available to the prosecution. There is no evidence known to the prosecution that the register of operations was prepared from information submitted by defendant SALZARULLO, and that such information omitted MACKAY'S name.

11. Without proof of some further connection between defendant SALZARULLO and the log in question it is evident that no trial jury could be asked to hold defendant criminally

accountable for intentionally omitting an entry thereon. Neither could a jury be asked to find the essential *mens rea* for the crime charged, the intent to defraud by concealing the commission of another crime.

    12.   No previous application has been made for the relief sought herein.

    13.   Under the foregoing circumstances it would be highly improbable that the People could establish the guilt of this defendant beyond a reasonable doubt and accordingly the People respectfully move this Court for a dismissal of Indictment Number 2050-77 as to defendant, LORNA SAL-ZARULLO, in furtherance of justice pursuant to Criminal Procedure Law section 210.40.

_____

PATRICK HENRY
District Attorney of Suffolk County

Sworn to before me this
19th day of June, 1978.

_____

JOB DESCRIPTION

TITLE:

Operating Room Secretary

FUNCTIONS:

(1) Knows policies, rules of Operating Room.
(2) Handles incoming and outgoing communications in Operating Room. Refers all staff personal calls to Supervisor.
(3) Books urgent cases excluding emergency procedures.
(4) Calls doctors' office to confirm date and time on tentative bookings taken by evening or night Supervisor, after 9:00 A.M.
(5) Processes requisitions and forms to other departments as required by the Operating Room Supervisor.
(6) Calls X-ray technicians when they are needed in the Operating Room.
(7) Runs errands to Laboratory for blood, X-ray and other departments whenever necessary.
(8) Takes doctors' messages when they are being paged.
(9) Records operations in Operating Room log book in a legible manner.
(10) Keeps doctors informed if there is any change in Operating Room time.
(11) Completes charge slips and brings same to cashier's office at end of day.
(12) Types Operating Room schedule and distributes same to the nursing units and other departments.
(13) Keeps temperature and humidity books.
(14) Submits time schedules to Nursing Office.
(15) Processes time cards on Monday mornings.

RESPONSIBLE TO:
OPERATING ROOM SUPERVISOR.

EXHIBIT A

JOB DESCRIPTION

TITLE:

Operating Room Supervisor

DEFINITION:

Registered Professional Nurse who under direct supervision of the Director of Nursing Service is responsible for the organization, management and direction of the Operating Room and Recovery Room.

QUALIFICATIONS:

Supervisor should be a Graduate of an accredited School of Nursing and be currently registered in the state. She should have had experience as a Staff Nurse, Assistant Head Nurse and Head Nurse. She should demonstrate good leadership, managerial ability, good sound principles of administration and supervision. Ideally, she should have completed a postgraduate course in Operating Room Technique, Administration and Supervision.

FUNCTIONS:

1) Assumes responsibility for overall supervision of all cases booked in the Operating Room and patients entering the Recovery Room.
2) Is responsible for Operating Room rules being enforced.
3) Keeps Surgical Control Cards current.
4) Provides for effective distribution and utilization of personnel in the Operating Room.
5) Keeps the Director of Nursing Service informed of reportable situations.
6) Directs activities of Professional and Non-professional Nursing personnel.

7) Directs procurement of supplies and equipment and maintains same.
8) Interprets hospital policies and procedures.
9) Promotes observance of Administrative and technical procedures according to established policies.
10) Directs in guidance and staff development.
11) Participates in committee work and conducts jointly with the Assistant Supervisor.
12) Supports and participates in In-service Education programs.
13) Promotes harmonious relationships with nursing units and between hospital departments.
14) Solves any problems that may occur with department heads and refers any recurrent problems to the Director of Nursing Service.
15) Is cognizant of the legal aspects of nursing, demonstrating this in her assignments, supervision and teaching.
16) Prepares weekly time schedules, monthly call lists and submits same to the Nursing Office.
17) Supports and promotes the Nursing Education Program of Smithtown General Hospital, the B.O.C.E.S. School of Practical Nursing, Central Islip School of Nursing and SUNY at Stony Brook.

RESPONSIBLE TO: Director of Nursing Service.

October 1975

EXHIBIT B